# THE GREEN FOODS BIBLE

## Could Green Plants Hold the Key to Our Survival?

David Sandoval

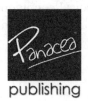

publishing

publishing

Published by Panacea Publishing, Inc.
PO Box 29004, Santa Fe, NM 87592
(877) 335-2683
www.PanaceaPublishingInc.com

ISBN-978-0-9914700-1-3 (Panacea Publishing, Inc.)

LCCN: 2015937472

# DEDICATION

I dedicate this book to all of those who take the time to reflect on the information contained within and to apply it to improve their lives and the lives of others.

# ACKNOWLEDGEMENTS

As a researcher interested in finding out the truth about how the body could rejuvenate and heal itself, I have been truly blessed to have studied with and be inspired by some of the most respected personalities in the field of alternative medicine, including Ann Wigmore, the mother of wheatgrass therapies and the greatest proponent of living foods. She showed me that one person's selflessness and love for others could change the world. She was like Mother Theresa, helping people find dignity and hope in their most desperate and needy time. She was my mentor, even if she never knew it. Rest in peace Ann. You inspired millions and I will always love you!

To Dr. Bernard Jensen, father of iridology and prostate cancer survivor, who coined the phrase, "If you are green inside, you are clean inside." Working with him in his last couple of years was like being the last person allowed in a library of wisdom the night before it closed forever. I kept wishing for more time, but perhaps my most important work with Dr. Jensen was convincing him to reconcile with his estranged son weeks before his passing. Thank you, Dr. Jensen, for your contributions to my understanding of disease and for the chance to help someone who has helped so many. You are missed.

To Dr. Herbert Pierson, former researcher at the National Cancer Institute. I never actually met Dr. Pierson, but in dozens of hours of phone discussions we found a kinship and brotherhood in arms. I first heard about Dr. Pierson from the National Cancer Institute, when a writer from Inc. Magazine told me that he respected my work and referred to me as one of the world's leaders in phytonutrient products. (Dr. Pierson initiated the functional food studies that proved foods fight cancer and disease.) Dr. Pierson died far too young, falling victim to a genetic form of terminal cancer that he could not overcome. So for everyone who has benefited from this knowledge, we have Dr. Pierson to thank. You, Doctor, are truly one of my heroes.

To Kelly Morehead, green food advocate, husband, father, and friend. Kelly also died too young, a victim of a cancer of the blood. When informed of his death, I read these words written in his last days—to the best of my recollection, Kelly wrote,

> "If you wish to say goodbye to me, do not sit on a plane to come to my funeral or send flowers grown in hothouses, since these use fossil fuels that deplete the ozone. Don't send cards or gifts that are made from trees or require Air Mail delivery. Instead, walk to the store or turn off a light you're not using, plant a tree or smile at a stranger. Do something to make this world a better place for our children, and then I can rest in peace."

So to Kelly I want to say, not a day goes by that I do not remember these words.

To my grandfather, who taught me that I could do anything despite the fact that he had come to America a poor immigrant. "A half-truth," he told me, "is just another name for a whole lie," along with his admonition that God gave me two ears and eyes and only one mouth, so listen and observe more than you talk! And Gramps had people using electric vehicles over 30 years ago...

To my father, Roman, whose early death left me unable to thank him for constantly pushing me to read, I hope I have made you proud.

To my mother, Mary Anne, whose faith in God helped her to overcome a difficult life and many maladies, reminding us that healing begins in the mind and spirit.

But mostly, I want to thank my daughter, Chloe. She is my inspiration to live and the source of my greatest joy. She has had to learn to share me with the world, and her understanding allows me to press ahead secure in the knowledge that the love we have for each other will endure.

In closing, while all of these people inspired me to write this book, it must be said that my co-workers' prodding and pressing pushed me to actually do it...and their constant support, hard work, and dedication have given me the strength to pursue my visions and dreams. So thank you to Amy, Cristina, Crystal, Debbie, Erin, Georgia, Gerry, Heather, Heidi, Marco, Martina, Michael, Nora, Tom, David Litt, Rodney, Noah, Fern, Jenny and the more than 100 employees and thousands of supporters worldwide. We have a big job to do, and the world is counting on us!

# CONTENTS

Foreword    xi

Introduction    xvii


*Chapter One    1*

Don't Just Survive: Thrive

*Chapter Two    15*

Chlorophyll Could Save the World: The Healing Power of Green

*Chapter Three    34*

Our Current State of Disease—And How Green Foods Can Heal Us

*Chapter Four    63*

Cereal Grasses

*Chapter Five    85*

Micro Algaes, Spirulina & Chlorella

*Chapter Six*    *103*

Cruciferous Vegetables, Leafy Greens, & Sprouts

*Chapter Seven*    *133*

Sea Vegetable Salad

*Chapter Eight*    *147*

Red is the New Green

*Chapter Nine*    *159*

Food Is More Than the Sum of Its Parts


Resources    206

References    211

Index    221

# FOREWORD

Can the blood of plants, chlorophyll, and its vast array of unique blocking, suppressing and repairing agents, be the key to survival of the human race?

Many people know that we should eat more greens, but, whether it is kale or watercress, there are far too many Americans who take a pass when it comes to eating them. *The Green Foods Bible*, David Sandoval's comprehensive and up-to-date guide, clearly explains why superfood should be consumed by anyone concerned with their health, because without sufficient green vegetables, optimal health can be elusive.

The need for superfoods and nutritional supplementation has never been greater than it is today. Our foods simply do not have the same nutritional value they once did. If you have bitten into a peach or a tomato purchased from a national grocery chain lately, the reason is clear. You surely noticed that these juicy foods were not like the fresh treats you once savored from your grandmas' trees, farmers' markets or roadside country vegetable stands. Those of us who live in large cities at a distance from growing fields have come to accept beautiful, but tough-skinned and nearly juiceless fruits and vegetables, with little flavor and even less nutrition, as a way of life. Our fresh food products are altered and engineered to have durable, thick skin for rough cross-country transit. They were picked well before the peak of ripeness in order to endure the sorting, washing, packaging, and trucking they must undergo before appearing in our local groceries.

Since former Surgeon General C. Everett Koop proclaimed the relationship of poor diet to disease, we've come to accept his now famous "5-A- Day" minimum recommendation for daily fruit and vegetable intake as somehow optimal for nutrition and health. As sound as this bottom-line figure is, most people are not getting even this minimum level of the vital nutrients they need in their daily diet. But in my opinion, as well as that of an increasing number of nutritional scientists, most of us need at least 12 servings a day of vegetables and fruits. Unfortunately, few of us are able to consume such a volume, let alone afford it. It has thus become far more practical to make up for our nutritional deficits by supplementing with concentrated and convenient sources of plant-derived foods.

As a specialist in integrative cancer treatment, I have long considered nutrition a key component in the prevention and treatment of disease and have found that green foods play a significant role in effective nutritional interventions. At the Block Center for Integrative Cancer Treatment in Evanston, Illinois, we utilize therapeutic nutrition and nutritional pharmacology as essential components of a comprehensive approach to combat and recover from malignant disease. After 26-plus years of developing personalized programs for cancer patients, I've come to understand that, much like the condition of the soil impacting nutritional health, a set of specific factors in the body's biochemical environment may impact tumor growth. My clinical experience has been confirmed by a growing body of scientific research that indicates that cancer therapy can be improved when we focus not only on eliminating the tumor, but also on favorably altering the biochemical climate that encourages tumor invasion and metastasis. This includes the deliberate use of nutrients, which, by correcting various key biochemical processes such as oxidation and inflammation, work as an important cancer treatment strategy and for prevention as well. In fact, in our clinic, with patients receiving individualized integrative interventions, we frequently see improved treatment tolerance, diminished side effects, and better outcomes than might have been expected. At the center of such interventions is the use of green foods. Green foods are not only profoundly nutritious, they provide therapeutic value and are also highly digestible and easy to use. Early in my clinical practice, I saw that combining conventional and complementary treatments into an individualized integrative program could have a synergistic and thus more effective clinical result. Since the primary goal for every cancer patient is to reduce the tumor burden while fortifying the body, we believe this integrative approach to be the best way to survive and thrive with a cancer diagnosis. Underlying our entire clinical program, however, is a basis of excellent nutrition. Core to the program is a whole foods, plant-based diet, a regimen of whole grains, vegetables and fruits, nuts, seeds and healthy oils, as well as plant proteins and specific animal proteins high in omega-3 fatty acids that counter the cancer-promoting inflammation from unhealthful fats.

Also integral to the nutrition program is therapeutic supplementation. With an optimal diet at the core, I advise a whole foods concentrate—yes, a super green drink. I advise each and every patient under my care to consume an assortment of green vegetables including crucifers, broccoli, carotenoid-family veggies, sprouted seeds, leafy greens, and other power-house, phytochemical rich plant foods. Since green foods are particularly important for my cancer patients battling disease, how much more so are they for those of us trying to prevent cancer in the first place. I especially urge my cancer patients, who may suffer from considerable oxidative stress, reduced appetites, and gastrointestinal disturbances during treatment or with advanced disease, to use this life-giving concentrate, critical to promoting good health through antioxidant protection and optimal vegetable intake. With green foods and our green drink as a foundation, we individualize a regimen of specific herbs, nutrients and other natural medicines to reinforce a cancer-fighting environment while addressing a range of issues and problems faced by cancer patients.

But patients with cancer are not the only ones for whom we recommend green food concentrates. Many of our patients are interested in disease prevention, and for these patients the phytochemicals in green drinks can also provide strategic nutrition. Consider the following scientific findings:

- Glucoraphanin in broccoli sprouts decreased oxidative stress in the heart and kidneys, reduced inflammatory cells, and lowered blood pressure in a recent lab study.

- Isothiocyanates in collards, bok choy, kale, and mustard greens inhibit cancer initiation and promotion.

- Dithiolthiones in broccoli, cabbages, kale, and collards trigger the formation of enzymes that block carcinogens from damaging a cell's DNA and inhibit the cellular processes involved in early and late stages of cancer cell production.

- High-lycopene tomato extract can reduce blood pressure in hypertensive subjects.

- Carotenoids in carrots, squash, and yellow peppers inhibit tumor growth and retard the development of cancer cells already exposed to carcinogens.

- Lutein in greens such as kale and spinach, as well as broccoli, plays a critical role in helping prevent age-related macular degeneration, an eye disease that steals the vision of many elderly people.

- Folic acid in asparagus, lima beans, and beets may help prevent chromosomal damage associated with the subsequent development of cancer.

- Greens, green drinks, and vegetable concentrates can benefit us all. We are each at risk of losing our health to the onslaught of free radicals, pro-inflammatory chemicals, and from exposures like pollutants and the junk food indiscretions of our youth. By making high levels of vegetable intake one of your key nutritional strategies, you can help protect yourself from these dangers and gain longevity at the same time.

By focusing on GREEN, David Sandoval has struck nutritional GOLD. His *Green Foods Bible* is a must read for each of us and is fundamental to our nutritional needs. Green foods and green drinks are a first step to buying back your health. It is assurance and insurance for your future and will help you bank the nutrients vital to optimal health!

Said simply, *The Green Foods Bible* is an excellent resource for anyone serious about improving their health and vitality.
—*Keith I. Block, M.D.*

Medical & Scientific Director, Block Center for Integrative Cancer Treatment and the Institute for Integrative Cancer Research and Education; Evanston, Illinois Director, Integrative Medical Education; University of Illinois College of Medicine; Chicago, Illinois Editor-in-Chief of *Integrative Cancer Therapies*, Sage Science Press Member, Editorial Board for Physician Data Query (PDQ), Cancer Complementary and Alternative Medicine (CAM); National Cancer Institute

# INTRODUCTION

Several years back, I began to notice a disturbing trend in the lives of the people I cared about. In increasing numbers, the people I loved were complaining of low energy, poor digestion, overweight, diabetes, arthritis, and dozens of other major and minor ailments.

My efforts to help make a difference in their lives and their health led me down a fascinating, fulfilling and challenging path. I learned about the benefits of a lifestyle that emphasizes raw, enzyme-rich food as well as the traditional healing practices from virtually every corner of this planet where thousand-year-old knowledge became profound in a modern world desperate for answers.

I have devoted over two decades of my life to discovering foods that heal and making them available in their purest possible, non-crossbred, wildcrafted forms. The foods that I seek are designed by nature to be especially easy to use and assimilate. The thousands of lives that I have been able to improve and the renewed hope that people feel is the fruit of those efforts, and my pride and joy.

The foods I recommend are unprecedented in their potency, purity, and in the complexity of their contribution to your body's well-being.

Within 90 to 120 days of embracing the knowledge revealed in these pages, you will feel your body awaken and thrive as it never has before.

If you believe that you are currently "healthy" and are looking for ways to stay that way, you have come to the right place. The powerful effect of "superfoods" that you will learn about in this book can take you from a state of average health into a stratospheric realm of energized well-being and resistance against illness. If you are basically healthy but often tired, coping with a lot of stress, susceptible to every cold or other bug that passes through your town, or just wish you had a bit more vim and vigor, my recommendations will give you that and more.

If you are currently challenged by illness or disease or fear that you may be in the future, you need to find an integrative doctor with qualified help. I have seen very sick people transformed by the powerful effect superfoods have on their body's ability to heal themselves from even the most dreaded conditions.

There is no safer approach to getting well than nature's approach, and that is the approach outlined here. I call it **Plant Based Nutrition Program**, and it involves tapping into the *phyto*chemistry (*phyto* is the Greek word for plant) that took nature millions of years to perfect.

In nature, every plant encounters enemies that would make them weaker or destroy them. The constant battle to survive and perpetuate various species becomes a testing ground or living laboratory that produces billions of chemical reactions every second of earth's existence. Over millions of years, any plant that could not resist bacteria, fungi, viruses, radiation, heat, cold, and pathogens of every imaginable form, simply disappeared. The plants that remain have each devised their own unique and powerful methods of resisting and defending themselves against these influences. Over the last 40,000 years, humans have identified the super-stars of the plant kingdom. These "super" foods contain powerful natural compounds that make them invaluable to not only the plant but the human body's ability to resist and defend itself against diseases.

We are specifically aspiring to cultivate and preserve the most powerful foods from around the world in an unspoiled, pure, and biologically active form, making access to these important tools more possible than ever before.

Whether you start out in sickness or in health, when you utilize these foods in your life, the aging process slows down. The physiological functions that support the blocking, suppressing, and repairing of your cells will be optimized. Your risk of cancer, heart disease, emphysema, diabetes, obesity, immune suppression, and Alzheimer's disease will fall, and you will drop excess weight effortlessly. Your skin will glow. Allergies and gastrointestinal complaints will dissipate. Health problems that have defied all mainstream medical treatment will be either eliminated or reduced in severity. Not because of a miracle, because your body is a miracle.

In my research and documentation of green foods, I've worked within a diverse group of cultural realms. I've worked to spread the healing message of green foods across Asia, Europe, and the United States, speaking, writing and educating others so they will be inspired to help me help all people improve their quality of life, remain free of disease, and achieve maximum longevity.

I work with cancer treatment centers, internationally renowned health food companies, celebrities, and some of the most popular personalities in the nutrition industry. My years of experience doing "Health Talk Radio" in NYC, heard all the way to Hawaii, gave me the unique opportunity to listen to people. I continue to write for magazines and to appear as a guest on radio and television, striving to inspire others to become as passionate as I am about living foods and their indispensable benefits for health and longevity.

I'm not a doctor. I don't have a Ph.D. in biochemistry, an M.D., or a degree in agricultural studies or ecology. What I do have, in abundance, is curiosity and enthusiasm, particularly when it comes to matters of the science of optimal health. When I realized the true benefits of green food, I went after the supporting evidence, much of it in obscure scientific journals. I devoured the information, and whatever I didn't understand, I found a way to figure out, calling upon a wide range of scientists and researchers.

I tinkered with these foods myself, learned to grow them and to formulate whole food supplements from them that packed all of the punch of the fresh, green living plants themselves.

I decided to write this book to show you exactly what it is I'm so passionate about—and how these foods can help you, no matter where you're at in life or health. I have seen the remarkable healing effects of green foods on people with cancer, diabetes, and every imaginable condition from acne to AIDS. I have even personally used green foods to transform and save people from death caused by morbid obesity.

No matter where you are coming from—under-nourished, overweight, sick, or trying to hold on to the gift of good health—this book will help you. You will find answers here. If I have done my job, you are about to become as passionate and enthusiastic as I am about life, superfood and green plants, and together we might just change the world, starting with ourselves.

My message is simple: You *can* transform your own health—starting with the food you put in your mouth. I guarantee it!

# *Chapter One*

## DON'T JUST SURVIVE: THRIVE

A dear friend's young daughter was diagnosed with a heart defect at the tender age of one year. In March 1996, at the age of nine, she was scheduled to undergo surgery to repair the defect.

He was already a believer in the healing power of green juices. Nine weeks before the surgery, he and his wife gave her two servings of Green Kamut, a dehydrated juice powder made from the tender, new leaves of organic Kamut wheat, each day. When the surgery was only 10 days away, they increased her number of daily Green Kamut servings to three.

My friend's daughter's medical team had advised him that she would be in the hospital for four to six weeks before they would be able to take her home. Once at home, they were told, they should expect her to be restricted to minimal physical activity for about four months. They had prepared themselves and her for this.

As she woke from anesthesia following her unusual and quite delicate surgery, the most amazing thing happened. She was being monitored closely in the intensive care unit. As the anxious parent sat beside her, she opened her eyes, and the first words from her mouth were not that she was in pain—

something that they were told 99 percent of people awakening from this operation would experience and express—but that she was thirsty! Her words brought out laughter throughout the entire ICU. To this day, Juan reports, she has not once complained of any pain from her surgery.

An evaluation by her physicians three days following the surgery led them to conclude that one of two things had happened. Her recuperation was progressing so rapidly that either something special within her body had triggered this quick recovery—or it was a miracle that had just happened before their eyes! "Because they knew that a body could not heal so quickly, they opted with the latter."

We, on the other hand, knew why his girl had healed so quickly. He attributed her rapid healing to Green Kamut wheatgrass juice.

Even more noteworthy, she did not spend anywhere near four to six weeks in the hospital. She remained there for only five days before she was given the "all clear" to go home. At home, she continued to drink the Kamut, and only 30 days later, doctors gave her no restrictions.

At the time Juan told me this story, he reported, "I am happy to say that my little girl is now very active. In fact, two-and-a-half months after her operation, she tried out for her elementary school drill team. She is now a full member of that team...She will always drink her Kamut, because she knows the true healing effects of this wonderful product."

Green foods heal. They heal on the individual level, as we've seen with this happy story of a young girl who regained her health. And they just might be a key part of healing an ailing planet.

## GREEN FOODS COULD SAVE THE PLANET

I've been thinking a lot about extinction lately.

Not about the extinction of owls or whales—but the extinction of the creatures that are more populous than any other mammal (aside, possibly, from rats).

That's right. You and I. Humanity. *Homo sapiens.*

Wikipedia defines extinction as occurring "when [species] are no longer able to survive in changing conditions or against superior competition." Typically, a species will naturally die out within 10 million years of first appearing on the planet. Some particularly well-adapted species have survived, virtually unchanged, for hundreds of millions of years without dying out.

Modern humans? Experts say we have inhabited earth for about 125,000 to 150,000 years—meaning we should be able to survive here for at least another 9.99 million years, give or take a few.

We may not, however, if we don't make some changes—and fast.

## ARE WE ON THE PRECIPICE OF EXTINCTION?

Some experts state that humans are currently in the second generation of a five-generation decline in our ability to sustain our species. I don't know about you, but I'm not ready to see humans call it quits so prematurely.

Evidence that we stand on the precipice of possible extinction goes beyond what we know about the population explosion and the sustainability of the earth's resources. It's getting worse!

Our food supply is over-processed, contaminated with multiple chemicals and compromised permanently by dangerous Genetically Modified Organisms (GMOs). At best, it lacks the nutritional potency necessary to support good health and sustain a species.

Fertility among North Americans is in dangerous decline. Sperm and egg counts among young adults are hitting unprecedented lows, and couples struggling to overcome infertility are increasing in number. This has been attributed to hormone-mimicking chemicals that have contaminated our food chain and concentrated in our bodies, disrupting the hormonal signals necessary for procreation. The higher we eat on the food chain, the more of these chemicals we're exposed to.

Research laboratories around the world are scrambling to untangle an ever-shifting web of drug-resistant bacteria, super-viruses, immune disorders, and deadly cancers that were unknown even 30 years ago. Millions of people are dependent on multiple drugs just to get through each day—drugs that, as we've seen, often pose significant dangers alongside their marginal helpfulness. Depression, anxiety, crippling fatigue, allergies, asthma, learning and attention deficits are all problems distinctly of the most modernized and prosperous parts of the world.

A lot of this has to do with what we eat—both with what our food lacks (vitamins, minerals, phytonutrients, fiber, and lots of other substances we have yet to discover) and with what it contains too much of (antibiotics, radiation, hormones, pesticides, herbicides, additives, artificial colorings, trans fats, artificial sweeteners, industrial wastes), and now GMO's!

I'd like to see *Homo sapiens* use our enormous brainpower, goodness of heart, and strength of will to pull back the reins on the environmental catastrophes that would spell our demise. We have the imagination and the intelligence to create a sustainable world. It was sustainable before we showed up and did so much damage, but I have faith that we have the ability to get it back there again.

A large piece of that puzzle involves major changes in the foods we cultivate and consume. As we change our diets in a radical way, we will change our own health in a similarly extreme fashion. We'll take in fewer of the chemical toxins implicated in damaging reproductive and immune health. We'll take in fewer of the foods that damage our arteries and set the stage for the growth of cancers.

From there, the microcosm of each person's health will translate to the health of the planet. Truly a win-win proposition! I don't mean to suggest that this is an easy transformation, however. Preserving our species on the planet goes back to our intelligent use of the resources it offers us. The food we eat is the most basic and fundamental of those resources.

Proper diet leads to proper health, and that proper health is the foundation upon which the future of humanity rests. Unfortunately, we are the only species capable of eating ourselves to death, and unless things change, we will succeed in doing just that!

Isn't that crazy? We are the most overfed yet malnourished people in the history of the world.

Since food is both a blessing and a curse, I've formulated my own approach to one of the most daunting challenges of the modern world, obesity; and as you might imagine, it's a Plant Based Nutrition Plan. I've seen this food plan transform a great many individuals from fatigued, fat, and forlorn to fantastically fit and full of life. It was even used to transform an 800-plus-pound ex-sumo athlete, Manny "Tiny" Yarbrough, back into his much more fit 600-pound former self. (Yes, 600 pounds; at six feet, seven-and-a-half inches tall, and about as solidly built as a person can get, Manny is a really, really big guy.)

## MEET MANNY YARBROUGH

In 1996, Manny "Tiny" Yarbrough was a minute late for the Olympic trials in Atlanta. He was disqualified from his most cherished dream: to be on the U.S. judo team at the 1996 Olympic Games.

He began his athletic career as a starting tackle on the varsity football team, and had played football for two more years in college. There, he discovered that he excelled at another sport: wrestling. Manny holds the *Guinness Book of World Records'* title of World's Biggest Competitive Athlete. At almost six feet, eight inches tall and over 500 pounds, he established himself as a worldwide ambassador for the sport of Japanese *sumo* wrestling.

A chance meeting with judo *sensei* Yoshisada Yonezuka swept Manny into the rarefied world of Olympic-caliber judo. After only a year of training, Manny was ranked fifth in the U.S. heavyweight division. In 1992, Manny got a call from Yoshisada about a sumo competition in Japan. Three days' training was all he got in this sport before he found himself competing in the first World Sumo Championships, and he reached the finals. This was where he became a celebrity. *Philadelphia Inquirer* writer Kevin Carter called him "the most important face in sumo, outside of Japan."

Manny appeared on talk shows, interviewed by the likes of Regis Philbin, Conan O'Brien, and David Letterman. He was always charming and polite, towering over everyone—a real gentle giant.

Fast-forward to those ill-fated trials. Then, Manny tipped the scales at a slim (for Manny) 550. He got depressed and started packing on the pounds. He stopped training, and soon topped the scales at 850 pounds.

Manny hasn't let go of the dream of being on the Olympic judo team. But his coach wouldn't train him until he was back to his fighting weight of 550 pounds.

## ERIC NIES TO THE RESCUE

Enter Eric Nies, celebrity fitness trainer, model, reality show star, self-described health nut, and MTV impresario.

When Nies caught wind of Tiny's tale of woe, he knew right away he wanted to help. Creating a Web site, a documentary film, and other media materials would allow Manny's story to help inspire others in a similar situation. Because of his popularity with teens, Nies hoped he'd be able to make the program accessible and attractive to a group that needed to wake up to this problem. Manny said yes, and the "Get Tiny" campaign was born.

In his own wellness program, Nies uses my green food products, so he called me to find out whether I'd like to get on board, helping to design a nutritional program for Tiny during his weight-loss crusade. Not only did I say yes to helping out with a nutrition plan, I also offered up my California ranch retreat as a setting for Tiny's transformation.

The program's kickoff, set to begin with an "official" weigh-in at Times Square, was delayed by one month due to post-9/11 security concerns. Then, finally,

Tiny stepped onto the scale amid shouted guesses as to what he might weigh. By then, he had already started the program, so his weight had "dropped" back down to 787 pounds.[1] That still left him with more than 200 pounds to lose.

## TINY'S PROGRAM

Our program for Tiny laid out fitness, diet, and supplement guidelines for this king-sized athlete. He began to eat a diet of mostly raw, organic foods, and to drink half his body weight in ounces of purified water each day.

I went shopping with Tiny and spent hours with him, coaching him on how to best feed his body for optimal performance and weight loss. Along with his diet, Tiny used several specialty foods. Some of these foods serve as the foundation of any Plant Based Nutrition Program, and others I recommended particularly to promote Tiny's massive weight loss. Prior to beginning the program, doctors told Manny that gastric bypass surgery was his only hope, and that trusting some nutrition guru's advice was dangerous. They warned that his weak heart, diabetes, sleep apnea and other conditions could not respond to diet alone...Sorry, Doc, wrong again!

On the program, Manny lost, on average, 12 pounds per week. More importantly, the fluid around his heart, his borderline diabetes, sleep apnea, joint pain, and virtually all other health issues disappeared, including high blood pressure and cholesterol. What was the basis of this miraculous Plant Based Nutrition Program? You guessed it. Green foods—lots of them.

## A WORLD APART FROM ISOLATED, SYNTHETIC NUTRIENTS

Concentrated green foods are unlike vitamin pills made from isolated, synthetic nutrients. They are *food*—food that can help to adequately nourish the

---

[1] His medical records showed his weight at 807 before he began to lose weight on the program we designed. Unfortunately, Manny's doctor had him on a diuretic that had him shed 50 pounds of water; in reality, his weight had started out at a whopping 857 pounds!

underfed and the overfed. Certain green foods are now being considered as the ideal answer to feed impoverished peoples in remote geographies.

Some of the green foods I study were the very first plants that grew on planet Earth (the algaes); others have been a key part of sustaining life on this planet for most of its history (the grasses); yet others exist in obscurity known only to those who have made it their passion, to dig a little deeper. These plants are the foundations upon which life on Earth is built and the answer to the growing health crises that virtually threaten ourselves and our planet.

I believe it is by studying our past that we can shape our future. By studying plants' ability to survive, we learn to survive as a species. We must pay attention to the gifts of nature and learn from them. We have the imagination and the intelligence to create a sustainable world, as long as we recognize where its greatest gifts lie and how to use them to the benefit of both ourselves and the planet we inhabit.

Changing our diets will result in changes in our health. Reducing the chemical burden on our bodies will result in reduced risk of heart disease, cancer, and the other chronic conditions that plague Western society. We'll be more in touch with our bodies and their needs, and hold those needs as more important than materialistic concerns. We'll feel more vibrant, energetic, and light, and this will translate to better attitudes, less conflict, more cooperation, and ultimately dramatic life extension and the fostering of wisdom.

Ideally, a renewed dependency on plants as our primary source of nutrition will renew our respect for and commitment to protecting the natural gifts of the earth. A more plant-based diet will reduce our dependency on drug- and chemical-intensive factory and monoculture farming, both of which use too many of our precious resources, disrupt ecological systems, and pollute the environment.

The microcosm of each person's health can translate to the health of the planet—a dietary version of that great old maxim, *Think globally, act locally.* Save your health, save your species.

I don't mean to suggest that this is an easy transformation, but it is remarkably clear and simple. Preserving our species on the planet goes back to our intelligent use of the resources it offers us. The food we eat is the most basic and fundamental of those resources.

Proper diet leads to proper health, and proper health is the foundation upon which the future of humanity rests the quality of our food equals the quality of our lives. Period. Amen. End of story.

## THE SYMBIOSIS OF PLANTS AND PEOPLE

Early Earth was a giant ball of molten rock, superheated by energy from the material collisions that created it. As our home in the cosmos cooled, this molten mass solidified. This process took about 800 million years.

Four-and-a-half billion years ago, the elements and trace minerals we depend upon for survival—the very stuff from which we are made, and that we need to consume in our diets—began to be laid down in the river beds of our newly created planet Earth. From those humble beginnings, the alchemy of life arose.

As the universe kept expanding and cooling, common particles began to form—nitrogen, oxygen, carbon, and the other elements—that became the building blocks of plant and animal life. Even when Earth became solid enough to stand on, with the formation of continental plates, it wasn't a very pleasant place to be. The atmosphere was filled with methane, ammonia, and other toxic gases.

The oldest life forms, *cyanobacteria*, appeared some 3.5 billion years ago. From that point for roughly a billion years following, the only life on Earth consisted of bacteria. We know this because of microfossil records, many consisting of the fossil remains of *stromatolites*, colonies of fossilized cyanobacteria that were once large mats of sediment-entrapping algae. Today, stromatolite fossils can be delicately sectioned to reveal ancient cyanobacteria and algae, perfectly preserved to the last detail. They are identical to forms of algae that are alive and thriving today—a testament to the hardiness, adaptability, and abundance of this plant form.

Around 2.2 billion years ago, the Earth had its first problem with pollution. This problem had to do with a relatively rapid increase in the level of oxygen in the earth's atmosphere. As cyanobacteria quickly multiplied across the globe, they released oxygen into the air, and in a matter of only a few hundred million years, the atmosphere went from 1 to 15 percent oxygen.

We think of oxygen as beneficial, and rightly so, but it does hold certain hazards. Oxygen causes *oxidation*, the process that rusts metal and otherwise transforms, breaks down, or destroys organic compounds.

In response to increasing levels of oxygen in the atmosphere, the evolutionary process came up with a new kind of cell: that which makes energy through the use of oxygen and releases carbon dioxide as a waste product. This process mirrors the process of photosynthesis, where green plants use the green pigment chlorophyll to make food from light, giving off oxygen. These are the cells from which we, and most other animals that inhabit the earth, are made.

In other words, without those first green cyanobacteria, we could not exist. Neither could newer types of plants. Within each plant cell exists an organelle called a *chloroplast*. This organelle is responsible for carrying out photosynthesis and making nourishment for the plant as a whole.

Here's the really neat part: Each chloroplast is actually a cyanobacterium, living within the cells of the plant! These microscopic cyanobacteria are the foundation of both plant and animal evolution. They are a sort of common denominator, an evolutionary link between animals and plants.

The evolution of other life forms—including fungi, animals, and humans—also is rooted in the cyanobacteria. Some 500 million years ago, cyanobacteria "moved into" certain cells that were the basis of these other life forms. The cyanobacteria would make food for the host in exchange for living quarters. Over time, this gave rise to the mitochondrion, the organelle found

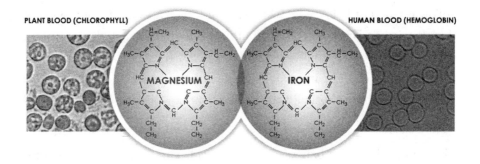

PLANT BLOOD (CHLOROPHYLL)        HUMAN BLOOD (HEMOGLOBIN)

in animal cells that is responsible for transforming food and oxygen into life-driving energy!

Most of the cells in your body contain mitochondria, and you have the cyanobacteria to thank.

**Today, algae are believed to comprise two-thirds of the earth's biomass,** forming a reliable foundation for the food chain that enables this planet to support its wildly diverse and plentiful tree of life.

At the root of green life on this planet is the process of photosynthesis—a process more complex than nuclear fusion or fission. Despite decades of study, science's understanding of photosynthesis is still incomplete. Through photosynthesis, green plants use chlorophyll to transmute the energy of the sun and the nutrients in their environment into their own growth, and so bring that energy to countless other creatures in the form of plant foods.

## THE BIRTH OF AGRICULTURE

When the first humans walked the land, they were basically meat-eaters who ate plants when hunger drove them to try everything that appeared to be edible. In those days, plant-eating was a risky business because it wasn't always clear whether a plant was toxic, poisonous, or nutritious. There was a good deal of trial and error before mankind figured out how to choose the right plants to eat. For tens of thousands of years we ate wild plants and fruits. Modern agricultural practices have narrowed our choices of plant foods down to a few of the thousands that exist.

Following the last Ice Age, in what was once known as the Fertile Crescent (Iraq, Syria, Turkey, and Jordan, all once much greener than they are now), agriculture was born, somewhere around 8,000 B.C. First, nomadic hunter-gatherers began to gather and consume, then plant and cultivate, cereal grasses. They began to build their villages around their food sources and abandoned the nomadic way of life.

First came wheat and barley. Then, animals began to be domesticated for meat and for heavy labor, as well as for their skins and milk. Cultivation of vegetables followed soon after. In Asia, about 7,000 years before the start of the third millennium A.D., rice, soy, and mung and aduki bean cultivation began. Around 5,000 B.C., corn, potato, sunflower, and squash cultivation began in what would become the Americas.

Grains were an enormously important part of primitive agriculture—they proved to be easily grown and safe to store for long periods. Grains remain an important source of calories for most of the people on the planet. It is estimated that two-thirds of the protein and calories in the diet of the average modern person come from grains.

The cultivation of grains ensured a greater volume of calories per person. It could support increasingly large groupings of people that evolved into civilizations. Agriculture concentrated the work of providing calorie-dense food, leading to greater leisure time, which paved the way for education, arts, and advances in technology. But, is a grain based diet good?

Anthropological and archaeological evidence does not indicate that agrarian societies fare better than hunter-gatherer societies in terms of health.

Hunter-gatherers are, on average, taller, better nourished, and suffer from less disease. Blood pressure in the people of foraging peoples runs a bit lower than in industrialized nations (averaging 105/65). More importantly, blood pressure does not seem to rise as these people age. Cholesterol levels are much lower than people in modern societies (averaging 125mg/dl), about the same as that for other primates, suggesting that values of this magnitude are "natural for primates generally. Obesity, hypertension, and diabetes are rare in hunter-gatherer societies. At any given age foragers tend to be about one-third more aerobically fit than Westerners. They almost never develop atherosclerosis, with the resulting heart attack, congestive heart failure, and sudden cardiac death. The incidence of cancer among hunter-gatherers is a difficult subject, but clearly they have benefitted from lower fat intake, lower tobacco and alcohol use, and a greater amount of fresh and natural fruits and vegetables that are not laden with agricultural and industrial chemicals.

They lived longer than farmers and had a much more varied diet. While hunter-gatherer societies could not sustain highly dense population centers, this didn't turn out to be a disadvantage. Densely populated villages and cities were most vulnerable to highly communicable diseases that could turn into plagues.

Some anthropological sources maintain that the quality of life of hunter-gatherer societies was better than that of agrarian societies, that their risk of famine was lower, and that they did not have to work harder to feed themselves, despite common misconceptions. Hunter-gatherers' encyclopedic knowledge of edible and medicinal plants was often lost to societies that became focused on farming. (How many people do you know who could hunt or gather anywhere besides the aisles of a supermarket?)

Since processed foods became standard fare in the U.S. in the 1950s, limp produce grown in depleted soils, sprayed with chemicals to keep the bugs away, and picked too soon has been the standard fare found in most supermarkets.

In recent years, the diet-disease link has become part of popular consciousness as health research makes this link incontrovertible. More attention is being paid in the media to advances in nutritional research, and to the hazards of a processed-food diet. More people know today than ever before that many disease processes can be prevented or slowed down with the right foods. Unfortunately, with the incredible abundance of tasty, sugary, fatty, easy-to-prepare, addictive junk foods, making a real shift to a green diet is not easy.

According to research surveys from 1997, some 74 percent of Americans did not meet the government standard for intake of fruits and vegetables: five servings a day. And those figures included intake of juice, which is usually pasteurized and far from the enzyme-rich, living food that is a piece of recently picked fruit.

Today, the government is recommending seven to nine servings daily. It's too soon to know whether more people are following these recommendations than were in 1997. For now, consider yourself. Are you getting enough fresh vegetables and fruit?

If you're like most people, you aren't. And when it comes to these foods, more is always better. Have you ever sat back after a meal and thought, "Man, I shouldn't have eaten all that salad"?

## THE MODERN "MOTHER" OF GREEN FOOD

Even as so-called progress brought us to the point of some people not eating any fresh, organic, locally grown produce at all, thinking people such as Dr. Ann Wigmore were starting a positive backlash. She was an important pioneer in the movement to steer humanity back towards its living green roots. Thanks to her persistence and convictions, being green got a little bit easier.

On a more personal note, Ann Wigmore was my mentor, teacher, and model, giving me the springboard from which I launched my life as a health educator. Those she inspired continue to move her work forward today. Her crusade to reach as many people as possible with her raw-food and green-food diet lives on, through people like myself and others who have become convinced of the veracity of her work.

Dr. Wigmore is remembered by most as the world's foremost advocate of raw food nutrition. In the pages of this book, you'll learn a great deal about what she taught about the benefits of raw food and green juices, and about how to integrate the best and most accessible of her teachings into your life.

# *Chapter Two*

## CHLOROPHYLL COULD SAVE THE WORLD: THE HEALING POWER OF GREEN

I recall an experiment from high school science class that involved a mouse, an exercise wheel, a glass dome, and a lit candle. The mouse would jog along happily, but then the oxygen in the dome would quickly be depleted, causing the mouse to lose consciousness and the candle to become extinguished.

We'd lift the dome and revive the poor fellow, using a little "mouth to mouse" resuscitation, and then try the experiment again, only with a mint plant under the dome this time. Under these circumstances, the mouse could run and run without the oxygen running out, and the candle would burn itself down to the tabletop if we let it.

Although I didn't completely appreciate this concept in high school—we were too busy thinking about lunch and cars and girls to be truly awed by the mouse under glass—today I can see that this is a microcosm of the world. The byproducts of breathing, heat, and pollution are converted into oxygen by plants, and this gives us life under the big dome of the earth's atmosphere. The difference between life and death under that dome, and on our much larger but similarly fragile planet, is the presence of green plants. Chlorophyll literally transforms light into life.

## BIOSPHERE II

In 1984, a group of scientists and investors came together to make an astonishing dream into reality: to build Biosphere II.

Biosphere II was a man-made closed biological system that would include seven different biomes—desert, rainforest, swamp, coral reef, savanna, intensive agricultural area, and an urban area—under a huge, nearly airtight dome that covered a three-acre area in the Arizona high desert. Many animal and insect species were brought into this futuristic version of Noah's Ark.

In 1991, with construction and creation of the various ecosystems completed, nine scientists moved into the Biosphere to live and perform research for two years. All of their waste and water were recycled. Over 100 different compounds were constantly monitored to see whether the project was successful—whether they were creating a sustainable, productive, non-polluting place that could sustain plant, animal, and human life.

The project was designed to earn revenue as a tourist attraction, and through the development of technologies, for example, devices for monitoring environmental variables, controlling pollution, recycling, or growing better crops. It provided an opportunity for research that would help humans have a less damaging impact on the planet, and to help heal the damage that has already been done. And a successful Biosphere project could, theoretically, be used as a model for a space station—a place of residence for humans on the moon or beyond.

Roy Walford, M.D., the Biosphere II physician who spent two years in that structure, made some fascinating discoveries of his own. He and his co-Biospherians ate a mostly vegetable diet with some meat and whole grains, almost all grown through their own labors. There was no processed, pre-packaged food to be found.

They lost an average of 16 percent of their body weight. Their blood pressure and blood cholesterol levels fell, and overall their health dramatically improved.

## WILL ALGEA HEAL THE PLANET?

Today, Columbia University is doing experiments with smaller closed systems in this giant desert laboratory. One researcher, Ed Glenn of the University of Arizona, is studying the effects of rising carbon dioxide levels—which, as you probably well know, is a major environmental problem today because of $CO_2$ emissions in exhaust and industrial wastes—on the growth of algae and seaweed, using the million-gallon tank that once housed a micro-ocean. His research is contributing to hopes that bursts of algal growth in the world's oceans could help to keep $CO_2$ levels in check.

That's right. Not only might we have chlorophyll-rich plants to thank for starting the evolutionary process that made us and every other creature on the planet, they could also slow down the ozone-depleting greenhouse effect.

And let's not forget that the green plants heal another kind of ecosystem: the one that comprises each individual human body.

## CAN GREEN FOODS HEAL YOU?

Anne's 73-year-old mom called her one day, saying she had almost run out of her green drink. She needed more, she told Anne, because she felt super, and didn't want to go back to feeling the way she had before she started following my advice. Anne's interest was piqued, so she tried it too. Soon, both mother and daughter were taking the green food religiously.

For years before that time, Anne had terrible allergies each spring—a common problem in Virginia, where she lives. She would start out with headaches as soon as the flowering trees sent out their blooms. Then, she inevitably faced sinus infections, then doctors' visits, then medicine, medicine, and more medicine. She started the green food program in the springtime, and since starting it, did not need a single pill for her allergies! Anne and her mom both feel it keeps their bodies clean. They love the peace of mind they experience when they know they're getting the daily greens required for good health.

The experience of Anne and her mom reflects a long history of Naturopathic applications for green plants. The earliest herbalists, Biblical alchemists, tribal medicine men, traditional Asian herbal medicine practitioners, and modern physicians all extol the benefits of green plants as a dietary mainstay. We all know that plants have medicinal value, and that hundreds of modern pharmaceuticals are derived from herbs and plants growing in the Brazilian rainforest, Africa, and various geographies.

Unfortunately, those drugs developed from plants usually focus on isolating individual chemical elements and studying their effects on a specific disease in a laboratory setting. When this is done, we forsake Nature's wisdom in putting together dozens of compounds that work synergistically, in concert with the body's systems.

The rewards for altering natural substances to make synthetic drugs are less about healing than about another kind of green. Synthetic substances can be patented and companies can choose whatever the market will bear without fear of competition for at least 17 years. This can't be done with natural molecules.

As you learned in Chapter One, an important evolutionary link between us and the plants is chlorophyll, the photosynthetic molecule—a molecule that is basically plant blood.

The molecule that carries oxygen through the bloodstream and drops it off at the cells is called hemoglobin. Hemoglobin is a part of each red blood cell in your body. You'll understand its role in the body better if we trace the course of oxygen molecules from the outside air and into your lungs, where each hemoglobin molecule picks up oxygen and transports it along the circulatory system.

As we breathe, oxygen and other gases pass into the trachea and down through the bronchial tubes. At the bottom of the lungs, oxygen is filtered into the bloodstream through tiny sacs called *alveoli*. Wrapped around each of those alveoli is a network of delicate capillaries.

Because the concentration of oxygen in the blood that flows through those capillaries is lower than the concentration of oxygen in the alveoli, the oxygen diffuses into the bloodstream. Right at that juncture, oxygen combines with hemoglobin in the red blood cells. Hemoglobin passing through those capillaries is loaded down with carbon dioxide, which it picks up after dropping off oxygen at the cells. This $CO_2$ diffuses into the alveoli to be exhaled from the lungs. This is a major part of detoxification. Each time we inhale, we must "digest" the air, taking what we need in and eliminating what would harm us. The more effective our lungs are, the more oxygen gets into our tissue, and studies show that in an oxygenated environment, bacteria, viruses, and even cancer cannot survive.

Like rivulets flowing into streams flowing into rivers, the blood flows from the capillaries into larger and larger vessels, and then into the left side of the heart. The heart muscle pumps this oxygenated blood into the arterial system, which branches off into arterioles and finally into capillaries throughout the body.

Capillary walls are only one-cell thick and highly permeable, allowing oxygen released from hemoglobin to pass from the blood into the cells. Those same highly permeable walls also allow wastes to pass out of the cells back into the circulation to be transported to the body's cleansing, detoxifying organs, and then disposed of.

A main difference between hemoglobin and chlorophyll is that at its center, chlorophyll carries magnesium, and hemoglobin carries iron. They are structurally similar in other ways. This similarity has inspired some to call chlorophyll "plant blood."

Let's pause here to make an important distinction between chlorophyll and hemoglobin. While chlorophyll is powerfully health-promoting, and while it has been found to aid in improving the oxygenation of tissues, it isn't interchangeable with hemoglobin. They are structurally similar, but not identical, and have differences aside from the iron/magnesium atom at their centers.

You might hear or read claims that chlorophyll can, once in the body, release its magnesium and pick up iron, becoming hemoglobin. This has not been demonstrated, and does not serve to explain chlorophyll's oxygenating effects, which you will learn about in greater detail later in this chapter.

## THE STORY OF ANN WIGMORE

Carnivorous dogs and cats instinctively chew green grass when their systems are not up to par. Humans don't have that same instinct—at least, not most humans. Ann Wigmore was different.

Dr. Ann Wigmore was perhaps the world's best-known promoter of a diet composed primarily of raw foods, and one of its most respected sources of knowledge about how those foods can benefit us.

In Lithuania in 1909, Ann was born prematurely and abandoned by her parents. Her grandmother rescued and raised her, and taught the child what she had learned herself about the art of natural healing. During World War I, Ann watched her grandmother use herbs and weeds to restore the health of wounded soldiers.

After the war, at age 16, Ann moved to the United States to live with the mother and father who had abandoned her. She began to eat a typical American diet, and ended up first with colitis, then colon cancer. Headaches and arthritis also afflicted her.

Ann resolved to return to her original diet of vegetables (especially greens), seeds, and grains. More specifically, she began a regimen of live foods—primarily, wheatgrass juice and sprouts.

As her body healed, she had enormous cravings for anything green. She devoured green plants in their raw state. She used fresh green plants to make poultices for her gangrenous legs.

As a result of her new raw, living diet, Ann underwent a startling change in her health. Her injuries healed and her chronic disease symptoms went away. Her hair changed from gray to its natural darker color; her vitality soared. This led to her live-food crusade, which eventually instigated the founding of the Hippocrates Institute in 1955.

The first Institute was created in Boston, then others were opened in Florida, southern California, and Puerto Rico. Tens of thousands of patients were successfully treated in these centers for a wide variety of conditions—including hypertension, cancer, diabetes, obesity, asthma, gastritis, stomach ulcers, pancreas and liver diseases, glaucoma, eczema and other skin problems, constipation, hemorrhoids, colitis, diverticulitis, bad breath, arthritis, body odor, gum disease, burns, and anemia—over a period of several decades.

Dr. Ann Wigmore was a doctor in the truest sense of the word: a healer who never did more harm than good.

Tragically, in 1994, she died in the original Boston home of the Hippocrates Health Institute during a fire. She was almost 85 years old, having lived a long, mostly healthy life, against all odds. Clinics based on her teachings have continued to open throughout the world, with six U.S. locations and others in India, Australia, Sweden, and Finland.

The programs offered at the Hippocrates Institute involve a diet completely made up of organically grown raw foods, along with fresh wheatgrass, vegetable, and fruit juices. They focus on the importance of living in harmony with nature and calming the mind in health and healing. Exercise, juice fasting, homeopathy, one-on-one consultations, and internal cleansing (including enemas and colonics) are other elements of the program.

I've heard and read some astonishing testimonials from people who have attended the Institute and who have adopted a dietary plan similar to the one taught there. People have been completely cured of the illnesses that have most confounded conventional medicine—including:

- Chronic sinus congestion

- Arthritis

- Fibrocystic breast disease

- Migraines

- Gingivitis

- Chronic yeast infections

- Asthma

- Tinnitus (ringing ears)

- Chronic fatigue

- Menstrual problems

- Fibromyalgia

- Multiple sclerosis

Some have also testified that the raw green, plant-based diet she promoted was a crucial part of their healing from various cancers—or, at least, to extend their lives and to feel well while fighting the good fight against those cancers. Robert Church, for example, suffers from mouth cancer, which caused him to lose his teeth and part of his jawbone. Unable to wear dentures, he lives on a liquid diet. Once he had discovered the eating program she developed, he was able to get the nutrition his body needed to feel stronger and healthier than he had in years.

Many of the diseases for which modern medicine has no cure are the result of complex, extremely gradual changes at the cellular level. Those changes are a direct consequence of a lifelong diet made mostly of processed, sugary, fatty foods. An intensive plant-based diet program is the fastest and most effective way to rejuvenate the body at the cellular level and to give it the raw materials it requires to rebuild itself and function more efficiently.

A plant-based, mostly raw diet is the diet for which human beings were designed. The standard American diet is, in comparison, toxic. (It's just as bad for our companion animals; Ann Wigmore advised a raw diet for cats and dogs, too.) A lifetime of eating toxic foods can gum up the body's works so badly that an intensive intervention like the Hippocrates Institute's is the most efficient and effective way to return the body to its natural balance.

While raw, unprocessed, organic, plant-based food should be a staple of every person's diet, a 100 percent raw, all-vegan approach doesn't work for everyone. In my work, I've tried to formulate programs that can boost the nutritional density, antioxidant capacity, and enzyme content of any lifestyle —so that even when you can't eat as wholesome or as raw a diet as you know you should, you can take comfort in knowing you're meeting your body's daily need for raw, pure, organic super food.

Dozens of healing substances can be found in green plants. One of the most studied of these substances is chlorophyll—the stuff that turns sunlight into energy and makes plants green.

# BENEFITS OF CHLOROPHYLL

Some of chlorophyll's properties include renewing damaged tissue, building blood, counteracting the effects of radiation, knocking out harmful bacteria, facilitating wound healing, increasing healthful intestinal flora, improving liver function and gum health, and triggering enzymes that produce vitamins E, A and K.

## CHLOROPHYLL AND ANEMIA

In 1936, Dr. Arthur Patek fed 15 patients with iron-deficiency anemia varying amounts of green chlorophyll rich liquids with their iron supplements. When the two were given together, red blood cells and blood hemoglobin levels increased more rapidly than with iron alone. Dr. Patek reasoned that chlorophyll must provide the body with building blocks necessary for the formation of hemoglobin.

In studies of sheep made anemic by bloodletting, feeding dry hay and green hay yielded quite different results. The sheep that munched green hay recovered their pre-bloodletting hemoglobin levels twice as rapidly as the sheep who ate dry, yellow hay. In other words, although hemoglobin and chlorophyll are not interchangeable, chlorophyll does have some effect on heme (hemoglobin) levels in the anemic body.

## CHLOROPHYLL, WOUND HEALING, AND INFECTION

In nearly every foot soldier's survival training, since the beginning of written history, they have been instructed that field wounds should be treated with crushed green leaves to create a salve to stop infections, excess bleeding, and speed wound healing. Scarring is reduced as well. Now modern science validates this.

For example: In an issue of the *American Journal of Surgery* published in 1940, Dr. Benjamin Gruskin—former Director of Experimental Pathology and Oncology at Temple University School of Medicine in Philadelphia—recommended chlorophyll as an antiseptic. Dr. Gruskin's experiments showed clear bacteriostatic (bacteria-killing) effects, especially against the severe infectious "bugs" that are often picked up in hospitals. He also pointed out that applying chlorophyll to a wound that had an unpleasant odor would promptly clear up the smell—great evidence that it was helping to eliminate bacteria. Dr. Gruskin also pointed out that chlorophyll helps to stimulate connective tissue formation, speeding up the healing of wounds.

Surgeon J. Norman Coombs, M.D., a colleague of Dr. Gruskin's at Temple, used chlorophyll to treat open wounds and deep infections that often develop around drainage tubes inserted into the abdomen or chest following surgery. These intrepid researchers found that open wounds could be treated with dressings soaked in chlorophyll solution, which could be applied as often as desired without any risk of skin irritation. These dressings, Dr. Coombs stated, "promote healthy granulation and wound healing...and hasten skin regeneration."

Carroll S. Wright, M.D., yet another professor at Temple, found topical chlorophyll helpful for the treatment of diabetic leg ulcers, rectal sores, vaginitis, impetigo (a bacterial skin disease common in children), and cervical infections.

Dr. Homer Junkin of the Paris Hospital in Paris, Illinois, used liquid chlorophyll as a treatment for advanced pyorrhea (gum disease). He found that this treatment caused the gums to "tighten up about the teeth," and that the previously abundant "purulent discharge" quickly dissipated.

On an intensive green foods program, people with chronic acne who haven't been able to cure their condition with drugs have been able to clear up their skin. Amy Lynn Venner was one such individual. She was always active and scored high grades at school, but had an acne problem that wouldn't go away. She spent thousands of dollars on dermatologists who prescribed everything from antibiotics to creams and injections. Fad-type cures advertised on radio and in magazines also ate up her money and offered no significant results. Nothing worked until she started drinking her body healthy with green food extracts. She wrote to me that on a recent trip to Asia, she was stopped several times by people who told her how beautiful her skin was. "I couldn't believe what a change these foods made," Amy wrote. "I have more energy and seem never to get sick. I recommend these foods to any teenager or young adult with skin problems who wants a real solution."

## CHLOROPHYLL AND SPERM COUNT

Research by Donald Fry at the University of California at Davis suggests that green foods contain important building blocks of sperm and can help to increase sperm count. Green foods may be useful in reversing infertility without drugs.

## CHLOROPHYLL AND SINUS HEALTH

Ear, nose, and throat specialists Redpath and Davis at Temple University have found that "green packs," inserted into the sinuses, helped to clear up congestion. The drying effect of the chlorophyll relieved congestion within an average of 24 hours in over 1,000 case studies who ranged widely in age (very young to elderly) and symptom profiles. Hay fever symptoms and sinus infections responded well to this therapy, too.

## GREENS, DETOXIFICATION, AND CANCER

Research by the Linus Pauling Institute at Oregon State University, published in the journal *Mutation Research* in 2003, found that chlorophyll suppressed cancerous changes in an animal model. The following year, Brazilian researchers obtained similar results in a study of cells treated with carcinogenic chemicals.

Research from the University of California at Davis suggests that chlorophyll may have neutralizing effects on the toxicity of the persistent pollutant DDT.

In a human trial, oral chlorophyllin treatment three times per day was shown to potentially reduce the risk of liver cancer in a population at high risk for the disease due to aflatoxin exposure. The researchers reported a 50 percent decline in levels of an aflatoxin biomarker in urine that seems to indicate a high risk for liver cancer.

Chlorophyll increases the resistance of guinea pigs to radiation and can help humans with thyroid cancer due to radiation poisoning.

However, green foods not only contain chlorophyll, but over 1,000 other substances, including lightweight proteins, nutrients, and antioxidants. Many yet undisclosed are a treasure trove of healthy power.

# CHLOROPHYLL'S BENEFITS THROUGH AND THROUGH

When you take a bite of chlorophyll-rich food—let's say, for discussion's sake, a few leaves of kale—the benefits start in your mouth and extend all the way through your digestive tract. They aren't limited to that set of organs, either, as you'll observe.

Most of us take our digestive systems for granted. If it's working properly, we don't even think about it. The truth is our digestive systems are always working hard to keep us alive and functioning. The GI tract never sleeps or stops to take a break, and we never have to put any conscious energy into keeping it going. We can eat onion rings and cookies and white bread, and our digestive systems somehow manage to extract from them the few nutrients they contain.

Your "gut" is, most simply, a disassembly plant. Except for fiber, your gut breaks down everything you eat into smaller components you can use easily. Then, these nutrients pass into the blood system in a form that your trillions of cells can use for body growth, energy and repair. This process of breaking down elements is called digestion.

Proper digestion is vital to our survival. Digestion is the process by which the foods we consume are broken down into useful nutrients and waste to be eliminated. Without a proper digestive process, nutrients will not be available, and toxic waste byproducts will not be eliminated.

The digestive process relies upon enzymes and probiotic bacteria that drive the chemical reactions we rely upon to remain healthy. Without proper enzymes and probiotics, we will suffer from constipation, arthritis, gastritis, allergies, yeast infections, obesity, acne, and body odor. Over-acidity will also contribute to hiatal hernia and the use of antacids that further decrease digestive effectiveness. Green foods are loaded with an abundance of digestive enzymes, and they promote friendly bacteria and neutralize excess acidity.

Most people mix many foods in one meal (meat, potatoes, sugary beverages and dessert). Unfortunately, our bodies are not conditioned or built by nature to handle this. So, they only digest proteins or carbohydrates at one time, but not both. This leads to undigested foods that may putrefy and cause decomposing food waste to poison the bloodstream. If you have been relying on an antacid to treat the symptoms of poor digestion, they may have dangerous side effects; they suppress the production of gastric juices for hours at a time, interfering with digestion. Ultimately, the diseases caused by toxic undigested food far exceed the discomfort of gas. Once again, green foods are the answer.

## BENEFITS OF CHLOROPHYLL IN THE MOUTH

The beginning of the digestive process occurs in the mouth, when your food is first broken down by chewing and is mixed with saliva—up to two quarts a day.

Chewing green leaves releases their nutrient-rich juices into the mouth. As they spread across the mucosa of the upper GI tract, many of those nutrients are absorbed directly through those mucosa. Bleeding gums, canker sores, gingivitis, and sore throats respond well to this inflow of chlorophyll-rich juices. Green juices have been found to slow the growth of oral and upper intestinal cancers—good motivation to thoroughly chew greens when we eat them. To take advantage of this anti-cancer effect when drinking green juices, swish them in your mouth a bit before swallowing.

Halitosis (bad breath) is caused by bacteria—in the mouth and further along the GI tract. Chlorophyll resists the growth of odor-causing bacteria in the mouth and further down, and so can help to control malodorous exhalations.

## BENEFITS OF CHLOROPHYLL IN THE ESOPHAGUS

After swallowing, the food is guided down 10 inches of esophagus and into your stomach. Here, green food helps to prevent heartburn and gastroesophageal reflux disease (GERD) by enhancing alkalinity (more on this shortly). Greens are extremely low in fat, too—another characteristic that helps prevent these common conditions.

Denise's story is a wonderful example of the benefits of plant-based nutrition on gastrointestinal problems. In 1994, she was diagnosed with acid reflux disease and began taking Prevacid. Shortly thereafter, her doctor put her on Nexium, "the purple pill." It really bothered her that she was taking medication on a daily basis (for seven years)—and at the time, she was only in her 40s. Denise tried going off the pills, but every time, her symptoms would return. Then, she read a book called *The pH Miracle*.

This book describes the acidity of the American diet; the risks of an acidic diet; and the benefits of returning to an alkaline diet and eating more green food. Denise followed the book's recommendation to drink green Kamut juice daily. She ate raw food for two weeks and did an internal cleanse. At the end of the cleanse, throughout which she kept on drinking Kamut, she had upper and lower GI exams. Her doctor was amazed and gave her a clean bill of health. He recognized that Denise had shifted to an alkaline lifestyle and encouraged her to "keep it up."

Denise discontinued the use of Nexium immediately, and has "kept up" the green drink for over five years at this writing. She reports that she feels better than ever. She wrote me, "Thank you, David Sandoval, for making the best green Kamut on the market. I cannot live without it!"

## BENEFITS OF CHLOROPHYLL IN THE STOMACH

The stomach has a volume of less than one-half cup. As you eat, the muscular walls of the stomach stretch and can hold about three pints of food and liquid. About every 20 seconds, rippling muscular contractions—*peristalsis*—squeeze gently with a churning motion, mixing the food with hydrochloric acid and pepsin, an enzyme. Once in your stomach, the greens you have eaten help to eliminate *H. pylori*, the bug associated with most stomach ulcers. *H. pylori* infection has also been linked to stomach cancer.

## BENEFITS OF CHLOROPHYLL IN THE SMALL INTESTINE AND LIVER

The small intestine is the body's longest organ (about 26 feet) and is an astonishing example of biological multitasking. It has some interesting similarities with the brain—the hormones secreted by the intestinal wall are very similar to the neurotransmitters made by the nervous system. Throughout the small intestine, nerves and hormones interact to orchestrate the passage of food through to the colon (large intestine).

The small intestinal lining also contains a vast population of immune cells that identify less tolerable foods. Depending on the level of tolerability of whatever you've eaten, the small intestines might do one of three things: 1) cause you to immediately vomit up the offending stuff; 2) cause bloating, cramping, or other discomforts collectively known as indigestion; or, 3) cause a paralysis of the small intestinal walls that allows your meal to pass very rapidly out of your body, mixed with plenty of water, a condition known as diarrhea.

Most of the green foods are well-tolerated, causing little to no GI distress. Some people have a bit of trouble with the crucifers (broccoli, cauliflower, cabbage, brussels sprouts), but allergic reactions or extreme sensitivity to edible green foods is virtually unheard of.

In the small intestine, food is further broken down into carbohydrates, fats, proteins, vitamins, and minerals, and those substances pass through the intestinal wall into the capillaries that surround it. From there, they go to the rest of the body.

There is some debate over whether chlorophyll is actually absorbed through the intestinal wall. Previously, it has been believed that it does not go into the circulation by this route—that it remains in the GI tract all the way through, with much of it being broken down by intestinal bacteria along the way. More recent research using sodium copper chlorophyllin (SCC) used a laboratory model to demonstrate that some chlorophyll is, indeed, absorbed into the bloodstream through the small intestinal wall, while some stays in the GI tract to bring its benefits further down the line.

Once absorbed into the circulatory system, chlorophyll promotes the liver's cleansing and carcinogen-neutralizing actions—specifically, increasing the action of the Phase II liver detoxification enzymes.

Researchers at the University of Hawaii found, during a year-long study, that adding chlorophyll to rats' drinking water significantly reduced the development of tumors in response to chemical toxins—particularly in the small intestine. Research by Dr. Alvin Seligman and others showed that chlorophyll complexes and certain breakdown products of chlorophyll have neutralizing effects on mutagens (substances that alter cellular DNA in ways that lead to cancer).

Chlorophyll appears to inhibit the absorption of dioxins from food into circulation through the walls of the small intestine. Dioxins are persistent pollutants found in many of the foods we eat, and they are known carcinogens. They are readily absorbed into the body and stored in fat. Earlier studies found that chlorophyll-rich foods in the diet increases the excretion of dioxins—the amount of dioxins that pass through the body without being absorbed.

## BENEFITS OF CHLOROPHYLL IN THE COLON

Whatever chlorophyll is left in your GI tract moves from the small to the large intestine, also known as the colon. Not surprisingly, it has benefits there, too.

The colon is sometimes called the large intestine; it's wider by far than the small intestine, but is only about five feet long. It begins in the lower right portion of the abdominal cavity and just under the liver, it makes a sharp turn and continues across the upper abdomen as the transverse colon, then makes another sharp turn downward. All of these sharp turns can prevent the efficient passage of waste out of the body, and can leave it to stagnate, irritate, and grow pathogenic bacteria. Green foods have a stimulating effect in the colon, aiding in the elimination of waste. Ann Wigmore advised ill people to use wheatgrass juice enemas to help facilitate colon cleansing.

One study from the Netherlands sought to understand why a diet high in red meat and low in green vegetables predisposes us to developing colon cancer.

31

They hypothesized that this could be due to the high content of heme (hemoglobin) in red meat. Heme is good to have in the bloodstream to carry oxygen, but it doesn't appear to be such a good thing to eat. In the GI tract of rats, heme is metabolized into a substance that is cytotoxic (toxic to cells) in ways that increase colon cancer risk—in part, by increasing the overly rapid formation of new colon cells.

The researchers gave rats either a control diet—normal rat chow—or a purified diet with heme added to it. Some of the rats on the purified diet got spinach or purified chlorophyll along with their heme. Then, the researchers measured the cytotoxicity of the rats' waste.

In rats that got only the heme-containing feed, the cytotoxicity of their colonic contents rose *eightfold*. Colon cell proliferation rate doubled. In the rats that got the heme plus the spinach or an equivalent amount of chlorophyll, both of these cancer-causing changes were inhibited completely!

Green plants enhance colonic *motility*—the contractile action of the colon walls that moves waste out of the body. Chlorophyll-rich plant foods are known to reduce *transit time*, the amount of time it takes for a meal to go from the chewing and swallowing stage all the way out of the body as waste. This is good preventive medicine for a long list of chronic conditions, including colon cancer, constipation, diverticulosis, irritable bowel syndrome, and flatulence. Green foods are often used as a sort of "intestinal deodorizer" because they reduce odors in the GI tract caused by the action of putrefactive bacteria.

## IN CONCLUSION: CHLOROPHYLL'S HEALING POWER

We'll continue to touch upon the benefits of chlorophyll, but there are a great many other chemicals found in plant foods that have comparably remarkable benefits. To fully grasp the scope of those benefits is to finally have strong motivation to shift to a diet rich in living green food. In a world filled with fast-food burgers, soda, and sugary goodies, this isn't an easy shift to make, but it is simple, and it works.

In the next chapter, you'll find out some common denominators or "usual suspects" of most of the chronic conditions that afflict modern people—some of which you might not have heard yet—and how green foods address those common denominators. I'll talk about specific health conditions and the effects of increasing green food intake on those conditions. Then you will learn about the various classes of green foods and how they can support optimum health and forestall most of the chronic disease processes that have become so common as to seem inevitable.

# Chapter Three

## OUR CURRENT STATE OF DISEASE—AND HOW GREEN FOODS CAN HEAL US

When I was six years old, I broke my wrist playing football. My parents couldn't afford a costly emergency room visit, so I was taken to see a family friend, Dr. Leonelli, who would give us a free X-ray. As I sat there whimpering on the gurney, I overheard a conversation on the other side of the curtain that separated me from the family of another patient that would change my life's perspective forever.

I heard Dr. Leonelli telling a woman and her kids that he was sorry, her husband had died. The heart attack he had suffered that day had been fatal. Never before—and never since—have I heard a wail like the one that came from that woman. She screamed, "But he was just sitting there, talking to us, and now he is dead!"

At that moment, I realized two things: One, that I didn't have much to complain about with my one broken wrist; and two, that people can look fine on the outside, but be sick enough inside to just drop dead one morning during breakfast. The seeds were planted in me then and that ultimately fed my life's work: helping people to promote their own health, inside and out, so they never have to be in a situation like that.

How about you? Would you know if you were dying on the inside?

If you feel sick, it might seem as though you *just* got sick. You felt fine before. One day, you started feeling bad, and then worse, and you feel like you've been ambushed.

In most cases, however, that health condition you now find yourself doing battle with has been slowly growing, expanding, occupying more and more of your body's energy and space—for weeks, months, years, even decades.

Inside the shell of your body, this illness has been gaining momentum, until finally it burst forth, leaving the fragments of your old life behind and dropping you into a new one filled with medicines, surgeries, side effects, and other indignities.

If you are not currently sick, terrific—but don't relax too much yet. Anyone living the typical overwrought American lifestyle and eating a standard Western diet is likely to be incubating some illness or other. You don't need to wait until you are diagnosed with a disease to take action to protect your health for the long haul. In fact, if you shift to a plant-based diet with quality protein from oily fish (if you are not vegan) and legumes, your vastly improved function and well-being may show you that you were ill and didn't even realize it.

Take the case of Dale, for example. He discovered some literature and tapes about the benefits of algae, and knew some friends using barley grass as a food supplement. He knew that the single most common item missing in the standard American diet was leafy greens. The testimonials he heard about these products convinced him to try "superfoods"—specifically, Green Kamut and other green drinks containing barley grass and algae. He didn't think he was sick, really, but wanted to take a proactive stance on his own health.

Dale had an immediate increase in energy. The green plant diet helped his digestion tremendously. He felt so much better that he started to tell everyone he could about these green food supplements, and convinced several of his friends to try them—with similarly excellent results.

This is a man who is nipping disease in the bud. He is reducing the chances that he will require the costly services of modern medicine.

## HUMPTY DUMPTY MEDICINE

The medical world is well-equipped to deal with the devastating transformation from apparently healthy to dangerously ill. Its technologies and techniques enable doctors to save the day. Or, in more down-to-earth terms, you could call it "Humpty Dumpty medicine," where all the King's men (the doctors) stand by to "put you back together again" when you fall off the wall.

What allopathic medicine is *not* well-equipped to do is stop the energies of a disease before it goes too far. Instead of trying to restore the body's balance—an approach embraced by traditional, natural medical practices like Chinese medicine and Ayurveda—modern medicine suppresses symptoms. This approach is something like putting tape on a leaky hose: a temporary fix that will only lead to more problems down the road.

Don't allow disease to incubate for years until it becomes powerful enough to kill its host (that's you). The responsibility of a phytochemical researcher is to seek out and to give people the information they need to interrupt these incubation cycles with (often) radical changes in diet.

The sooner we interrupt those incubation cycles, the better.

## START THEM YOUNG

Children are the most vulnerable of all to the perils of poor diet. The foods we give them during the crucial years between weaning and adult-hood will make a dramatic difference in the most basic functioning of their bodies throughout their lives. They are what they eat, and most kids are eating completely compromised food both in school and at home. And children don't have the sense adults have that they need to eat healthful things often, even if they aren't delicious. The wide availability of junk food, fast food, and highly processed treats makes a parent's job in funneling the right nutrients into their children even harder. Unfortunately, many parents are not even aware that "treats," "surprises," and comfort foods are harming their children.

Multivitamins and other nutritional supplements are a misguided approach to ensuring adequate nutrition, and many studies now reveal the false promise of chemically composed synthetic or isolated concentrated nutrients. Worse, many contain processed sugars, artificial colors and flavorings, and only serve to make parents feel better about the poor diets they will not or cannot change. And parents have to be extremely careful to give kids the right balance of nutrients. With some nutrients, too-high intake over a long period of time can be dangerous (particularly, vitamin A, vitamin D, and iron). Giving kids whole green food in the form of a shake is a much more holistic, safe approach. It helps them to learn that vitamin pills aren't the answer to good nutrition—it's real food. If you want a real natural multivitamin, check out the nutritional profile of spirulina.

Chris and Kelly were at a regional meeting when they got their first introduction to concentrated green foods. They had read about some of the ingredients before—spirulina, cereal grass juices—and were excited to try them. The drinks made with green juice tasted great to them, but what they were unprepared for was the reaction they got from their five-year-old daughter, Kaetlin.

Kaetlin's parents dared her to try the drink. She proceeded not only to try it, but to guzzle the entire glass of bright green juice. All in attendance were shocked! Chris and Kelly told Kaetlin that if she would drink a green drink every day, they'd never nag her to eat her vegetables. She agreed, and now everyone's happy. Mom and Dad know their child is well-nourished, and Kaetlin doesn't have to fight with her parents over how many bites of spinach she has to take at the dinner table.

## THE FALSE PROMISE OF MODERN MEDICINE

Optimal health requires that we pull away from dependency on over-the-counter (OTC) drugs and prescriptions and trust in the power of nature to heal us in all but the most extreme of circumstances.

The majority of pharmaceutical companies' most profitable products do little more than introduce more toxicity into our systems, in addition to causing often unacceptable or even life-threatening side effects—often conveniently requiring another drug to counteract the side effects of the first one. Green foods provide the foundation for true wellness and freedom from drugs.

Your body cannot be healthy without a balanced diet. And you cannot have a balanced diet without colorful vegetables and fruit—"living food"— and minimally processed.

As it has been established, foods that contain chlorophyll—and a host of other phytonutrients (plant nutrients) that will be described in more detail throughout this book—have potential for helping your body heal and prevent a wide variety of conditions, allowing us to reach our maximum longevity.

## YES, BUT WE'RE LIVING SO MUCH LONGER WITH MODERN MEDICINE...

Can we live to be 100? Or even 150 years old? Possibly. Statistics say we're living 30 percent longer than we did at the turn of the century. If this trend continues, it stands to reason that life spans of 100 and up to 150 should be realized within just a few generations...right?

Unfortunately, statistics lie. We aren't truly living 30 percent longer than we did at the turn of the century. In fact, we have come up with so many artificial means to extend life that any statistic relating to longevity certainly must first be measured against these phenomena. The four leading cases of death 100 years ago have dropped dramatically; infant mortality, the plague, the reduction of accidental deaths, war, and combined with the increase in medical advances that keep us alive by artificial means today more than compensate for this supposed decrease. Upon examining these statistics, it could be argued that life span hasn't increased at all. The clearest evidence is that the same percentage of our population lives to be 100 as way back then— no more, no less.

Let's assume that it makes good sense to extend each human's healthy life span, and to help them avoid costly, painful, joy-sucking infirmities in the last few decades of their lives.

What can we do to extend life? Believe it or not, it has been proven that in certain civilizations—some of them ancient—that people can and do live to be anywhere from 100 to around 125 years old, maybe older. If this is within the realm of possibility, why is it that men almost never pass the century mark, and why does only about 1 percent of the human population ever reach 100 years of age?

Numerous studies have been done to find out what contributes to increased longevity. Here's what they've found: The only sure way to increase your life expectancy, and the best way to halt or reverse the aging process, is through the consumption of nutrient-dense, low-calorie, *plant-based* foods. That means you need to consume a high amount of plants, fruits, vegetables, seeds, nuts, grains, beans, legumes, roots, and tubers. These foods are the key to a long, disease-free life.

## IT'S THE CALORIES

Why is it that a plant-based diet is the ideal diet to extend life? The reasons are many, but they all boil down to the simple equation of calories in and energy expended.

We typically consume far too many calories. Over consuming calories excessively accelerates the metabolic process, which in turn increases wear-and-tear at the level of each individual cell, as well as the level of the organs and of the entire body. Science knows for sure that this plays a huge role in shortening human life span. If we consume the ideal number of calories for our energy needs in any given day, then we will maximize our life span. That boils down to eating highly nutrient-dense food, and getting some exercise on most days.

It's absolutely clear that populations who eat more greens are healthier and more vital and live, on average, longer and more disease-free life spans. There is total agreement by researchers that phytonutrients prevent premature "death by disease." These phytonutrients are extremely powerful and work together so perfectly that no combination of synthetic drugs or supplements is comparable.

Green foods are an important addition to the day-to-day life of any person who's interested in optimal health. But they work best when added into a lifestyle that includes an overall healthy diet, stress relief, and an exercise program. Everyone can use green foods to help deal with today's unusually stressful lifestyles, polluted environment, or bring balance to a fast-food diet. You can make delicious blended drinks and snacks, and have these if you like even while sitting around watching TV for three hours a day. At least it will be the start of something better.

Every bit helps, but if you want to get the most out of green power, you'll allow those green foods to draw you into a holistic approach to your own health that will keep you out of doctors' offices and hospitals.

I've done a lot of research and lectured across the world, fueled by the desire to help people improve their quality of life and achieve maximum longevity free from disease.

Today I try to walk the talk of the "super foods lifestyle," and teach others that the road to health is paved with...plants!

## WE CAN'T DRUG OURSELVES INTO GOOD HEALTH

Open any magazine or newspaper. Turn on the television. Within a short time, you're bound to see advertising for a prescription drug.

These ads are so appealing: attractive people frolicking in flower-dotted fields (despite their hay fever); doing some athletic activity (despite their arthritis); or socializing happily (despite their chronic depression, social anxiety disorder, ED, or genital herpes). There's so much prettiness to see and hear while watching such advertisements on television or paging by them in a magazine that you may find yourself tempted to ignore the fine print about the drugs' risks. But, if you listen closely to the announcer's rapid-fire elocution of a long list of side effects that run the gamut from annoying to life-endangering, we would always ask "isn't there a better way?" We will not hear about natural alternative on TV, but we will see drugs, drugs, and more drugs!

So-called direct-to-consumer (DTC) advertising for drugs is so common today that you forget when it didn't exist. Actually, DTC ads for prescription drugs were against the law until the mid-1990s. In most countries, they are still illegal.

Here, they have contributed to a reliance on prescription drugs that is directly at odds with truly healthful living. This reliance has led to some "43 percent of persons taking at least one prescription drug during any given month, with 500,000 deaths each year attributable to drugs that are prescribed by physicians."

At one time, the pharmaceutical industry was the source of drugs that saved countless lives. Antibiotics and antimalarial drugs have played an enormous role in improving public health and prolonging human life spans.

But now, the drugs that sell the best are not the ones that truly save lives; they are the drugs that are used to treat chronic conditions—conditions that are believed by mainstream medicine to be incurable. A person who takes drugs for a chronic condition will, in the view of the medical mainstream, need those drugs for the rest of his or her life. And it estimated that 100 million Americans have at least one chronic condition. Add to this the many drugs used to control so-called "risk factors" for heart disease, including high cholesterol, type 2 diabetes, and high blood pressure. That's a lot of money going out of our pocket and into the drug makers' coffers.

The problem with prescriptions is that they control symptoms without healing the person. All too often, they cause problems themselves in the form of side effects.

At this writing, consumers are becoming ever more suspicious about the drugs that have been pushed on them, largely due to a series of drug recalls starting in the 1990s. Medicines that were supposed to be the next big best thing ended up having too many dangers to be widely used—or, in the case of some, to even be used at all. Drug makers have been caught manipulating study data and buying off research teams to ensure that they'd get results positive enough to earn FDA approval for their next blockbuster.

Fortunately, many people with chronic conditions don't really need to use drugs to control those conditions. With a dietary and supplement over- haul, these people may be able to do what the medical community can't— actually reverse a chronic condition and make themselves totally well again.

## HEALTH PROFESSIONALS USE THESE GREEN FOODS, TOO

Naturopathic doctor, herbalist, and lecturer Donna Bach has come to rely on concentrated green foods for virtually all of her patients. She appreciates the purity, potency, and variety of these foods, and finds that having them all on a few products she can recommend to patients is an amazing gift.

Dr. Jerry Schwartz of New York City is a clinician who deals with people's most intimate emotional and physical issues on a daily basis. He has come to rely on nutrition as an effective tool in his practice. He has called the availability of extremely potent whole food concentrates in a comprehensive program like my Plant Based Nutrition Programs "an important breakthrough." He goes on to say that "a diet properly balanced through 'power food' consumption creates a physical environment that allows mental stress to be relieved. Under these circumstances, I get a much clearer picture of the clients' entire psychological and physiological status." He recommends Plant Based Nutrition Plans to anyone "truly dedicated to self-improvement."

Even Dr. Keith Block, head of one of the leading integrative cancer treatment centers in the world (based in Evanston, Illinois), used green plant-based nutrition products to assist his patients in better tolerating and recovering from cancer-fighting drugs.

At the Block Center for Integrative Cancer Treatment, Dr. Block performs a comprehensive lab analysis evaluating nutrients, phytochemicals, and oxidative, inflammatory, immune and other markers that he has shown can be improved through a plant-based diet. Over the years, Dr. Block has had many patients outlive their expected survivals with various metastatic cancers. While he believes this is due to his personally tailored integrative program, he also points out that his clinical use of natural medicines and green foods is key to his patients' success.

## WHAT IS A CHRONIC CONDITION?

Chronic conditions are the major cause of illness, disability and death in the United States. It is projected that by the year 2040, some 160 million Americans will have a chronic condition, and that the costs of treating those conditions will reach or exceed 864 billion dollars.

## 'COMMON DENOMINATORS' OF CHRONIC DISEASE

Using drugs to treat chronic disease is like playing Whack-A-Mole. One little mole's head pops up, you whack it with a wooden mallet, and another mole's head pops out of another hole.

You're not doing anything about the mole problem. If the game didn't end, you could be there forever, whacking away.

Medical treatment of chronic disease usually involves one or more drugs targeted at specific symptoms. For example: Medical treatment of a person with heart disease often includes drugs to lower blood pressure, drugs to lower cholesterol and triglycerides, drugs to thin the blood, and drugs to help regulate an irregular heart rhythm.

## SOME COMMON CHRONIC CONDITIONS

- Arthritis

- Asthma

- Attention deficit/hyperactivity disorder (ADHD) and attention deficit disorder (ADD)

- Autoimmune diseases (Crohn's disease, lupus, rheumatoid arthritis)

- Bronchitis

- Cancer (not widely considered to be chronic, but included because it tends to recur and because it shares many of the "common denominators" I will discuss in the remainder of this chapter)

- Cataracts

- Depression

- Dermatitis (including eczema and psoriasis)

- Diabetes

- Hay fever

- Hearing impairments

- Heart disease

- Hypertension (high blood pressure)

- Orthopedic impairments (joint or bone problems not related to arthritis)

- Sinusitis (congestion, inflammation, and infection in the sinuses)

To see this list of medicines, you might think that each of these symptoms springs from a different source. The going medical wisdom is that they can only be dealt with separately, and that by controlling cholesterol and blood pressure and blood viscosity with medicines, we are doing all we can to prevent the clogging or clenching of an artery in the heart that is a heart attack.

The truth is that the symptoms of heart disease—and, really, almost any chronic disease—can all be boiled down to a few common denominators. They are:

1. Inflammation

2. Oxidation

3. Lack of alkaline factors in the diet

4. Lack of enzymes in the diet

5. Lack of trace minerals in the diet

6. Difficult or stagnant eliminative function

7. Toxic exposures

If we can apply our knowledge of healing foods and lifestyle changes to adjusting these factors—to bringing them within optimal ranges in our bodies—we can prevent virtually every chronic disease that afflicts our species. I have seen and been told of many instances where chronic diseases were cured and the body returned to radiant health with the help of a concentrated green foods program, because such a program addresses the common denominators of these diseases. In fact, I do not hesitate to say that green foods are the closest thing to a panacea, a "cure-all," than any other source, whether natural or from a scientist's laboratory.

This may sound outrageous or impossible to you, particularly if you have been struggling with chronic disease. Please keep in mind that if a disease has progressed past a certain point, permanent damage may have been done (sometimes, it's *iatrogenic* damage, done by the mainstream medical treatments that have been applied in efforts to help you), and a complete reversal may not be possible. Even so, you most certainly can improve your health and live a clearer, better, more energetic life with green foods than without.

What you are really doing by shifting to a green foods lifestyle is maximizing your own body's natural healing powers. The human body—and the bodies of animals—are designed to heal themselves. It's astonishing, really, how good these physiological systems are at fixing what's broken, as long as there aren't too many accumulated toxins interfering with or interrupting these processes which could also explain a lot since green foods eliminates those toxins!

The concept of many diseases being caused by imbalances is not new. Natural medicine has long sought to help people heal from diseases by identifying underlying factors that *predispose* us to ill health. In traditional Chinese medicine (TCM), these factors are referred to in terms of imbalances between yin and yang. By applying therapies to enhance one or the other, these complementary energies are balanced within the body, and health is improved. A TCM doctor does not wait for the patient to become overtly ill to begin addressing yin/yang imbalance; instead, he or she draws on extensive training and diagnostic techniques to tip the scales in the proper direction long before the patient is seriously ill.

In Ayurvedic medicine, the traditional medical practice of India, each person is seen as a distinct combination of three *doshas*—qualities of body shape and size, energy, and disposition—that can be appropriately balanced and manipulated with the right foods, herbs, and other therapies. The Ayurvedic physician can detect imbalances far subtler than those detectable through modern Western allopathic medicine, and can correct these imbalances through natural means before the patient is too far gone to come all the way back to good health.

In their own ways, TCM and Ayurveda—and every other healing modality that heals rather than poisoning the body with a barrage of drugs—deal with the same factors we'll now take a brief look at ourselves.

# INFLAMMATION

At this writing, the latest health news is, it seems, all about inflammation—or, more specifically, excessive, slow-burning, low-grade inflammation. It is believed to be at the root of most chronic health problems. It is also believed that there's no avoiding chronic health problems without addressing the inflammation issue. Medical tests, supplements, and special diets are widely recommended for the purpose of inflammation control.

This natural process is a function of the immune system, designed to enable the body to identify, target, and eliminate pathogens with the least possible collateral damage. A sprained ankle becomes inflamed—red, hot, painful, and swollen—and over time, the inflammation is cleared by the body's waste disposal mechanisms, and the ankle heals. An infected cut also becomes inflamed as the body's immune defenses are drawn to the area. When you have a cold, flu, or feverish illness, you might experience inflammation in various places in the body—the membranes lining the nose, or the respiratory passages, or the muscles or joints, for example. A fever is actually a full-body inflammatory response to infection.

I won't deny that inflammation is an important root factor in many chronic conditions, including the autoimmune diseases (rheumatoid arthritis, psoriasis, Crohn's disease, lupus) and allergies (nasal and skin). It has also been implicated as a contributing cause of heart disease (inflammatory factors contribute to the formation of plaques in artery walls), Alzheimer's disease, and even some cancers. Chronic inflammation is widely believed to play a role not only in nasal allergies but in asthma as well; it appears to enhance overall sensitivity to allergens and the body's response to those allergens. Pain that won't go away may also be hanging on because of an overblown inflammatory response.

Diet and genetic predisposition strongly affect the body's tendency to overshoot when it comes to inflammation. A diet high in processed and cooked foods, particularly those made from white flour, sugar, dairy, and meats, will push the body towards a more inflammatory state. This typical dietary pattern alters specific hormonal and immune-system pathways in the body that directly affect the inflammatory process.

A diet rich in vegetables, fruits, whole grains, and fish (for non-vegans) pushes the inflammatory balance in the other direction—food as a natural anti-inflammatory. We have good reason to believe that this will prevent age-related, degenerative diseases.

Some of these anti-inflammatory superstars of the food kingdom include some of the darkest pigmented plants including cherries, blue berries, pomegranates, which everyone knows about but now we are learning about spirulina, astaxanthin, and my new favorite green tea seed oil.

## OXIDATION

In the process of cellular metabolism, reactive singlet electrons called *free radicals* are created in a process called oxidation. A free radical is a molecule that contains unpaired electrons. Free radicals are also produced by the immune system when it identifies and eliminates pathogenic agents, and by the inflammatory process (which I'll tell you more about in the next section). Tobacco smoke and air pollutants increase the free radical burden in the body.

Imagine that each of your body's cells is a photocopier, responsible for duplicating itself. If there is a defect in the original, that defect is passed onto the copies made from it. Over time, more flaws appear, and each is passed down to the cells' progeny, until these "photocopies" are so flawed that they can no longer be read. These flaws are created by a process called oxidative decomposition—a gradual decay caused by the natural process called oxidation.

Like people, electrons prefer to travel in pairs; when one is "alone" it immediately looks for a new electron with which to pair itself, and will "steal" one from another "healthy" molecule. It might steal this electron from genetic material (DNA), cholesterol or other fats, or proteins— creating singlet electrons and new free radicals. A chain reaction of oxidation is set in motion.

Unless the chain is stopped by the action of an antioxidant—basically, an electron donor or receiver that gets electrons paired up again, a sort of sub-atomic matchmaking—damage can occur. This damage is microscopic, but it accumulates over time as damaged cells replicate themselves.

Most scientists who study aging and age-related diseases agree that excess free radicals are a major factor in the aging process, and in the development of the diseases we fear most: heart disease (caused in part by free radical attack on LDL cholesterol in the bloodstream), cancer (initiated by free radical attack on DNA), and Alzheimer's disease (believed to be caused in part by accelerated free radical formation in specific areas of the brain).

Antioxidants are the answer, but not just any old antioxidants. It's clear from the research that taking megadoses of antioxidant vitamins such as C, E, and A won't adequately control oxidation. In fact, taking too many of these antioxidants without proper balance can *increase* free radical formation. Why? Because all of the antioxidants work together, donating electrons to one another; if this doesn't happen, the antioxidants themselves can end up becoming free radicals themselves when they donate their own precious electrons.

We require the synergistic combinations of antioxidants that are found in very high concentrations in—yes, you guessed it—fresh, raw foods, particularly deep-green foods. As you read on, you will learn more specific, research-based information about the many antioxidants found in different varieties of green food.

## LACK OF ALKALINE FACTORS IN THE DIET

You may recall from a long-past chemistry class that acidity and alkalinity are measured on a scale of 0 to 14. At the center of this scale is 7, or neutral pH (the letters stand for "potential of hydrogen"). The pH is a measurement of the number of hydrogen ions. Human blood has a pH strictly maintained between 7.45 and 7.35, which means that in its natural state, it is slightly alkaline. Maintaining this alkalinity is essential for life; if blood pH goes outside of the range of 6.8 to 8.0 for more than a few seconds, coma and death will result.

Fortunately, the body has developed a lot of fail-safe mechanisms for keeping pH within these limits. Maintaining optimal pH with a diet rich in green foods isn't imperative for keeping you alive today, but reducing the amount of work your body has to do to control pH can make a big difference in your health over the long haul.

Control over the pH of the body is maintained primarily by the respiratory system and the kidneys.

Deep breathing alkalinizes the body by getting rid of excess carbon dioxide ($CO_2$). A person who breathes shallowly will accumulate extra $CO_2$ in the bloodstream. The $CO_2$ combines with water ($H_2O$) to form carbonic acid, and pH falls. This is known as *respiratory acidosis*. Respiratory acidosis is a medical emergency in which decreased ventilation (hypoventilation) causes increased blood carbon dioxide concentration and decreased pH (a condition generally called acidosis).

Carbon dioxide is produced continuously as the body's cells respire, and this $CO_2$ will accumulate rapidly if the lungs do not adequately expel it through alveolar ventilation. Alveolar hypoventilation thus leads to an increased $PaCO_2$ (called hypercapnia). The increase in $PaCO_2$ in turn decreases the $HCO_3^-/PaCO_2$ ratio and decreases pH.

The kidneys work to prevent *metabolic acidosis* by continually buffering acidity with minerals. Those minerals may have to be pulled from the body's stores in bones and elsewhere if the diet is consistently acid-producing. An alkaline diet helps to preserve those mineral stores for other important uses. An acidic diet is associated with kidney stones; as acid leaches minerals from bones, blood levels of minerals rise and any excess is deposited in the kidneys in the form of stones.

Acidosis can also result when blood supply to tissues is compromised, a common problem in people with unhealthy circulatory systems. When oxygen-rich blood can't get into an area to bathe the tissues, oxidative metabolism—the process where oxygen is used to "burn" fuel into energy— can't proceed efficiently. Instead, a less efficient, non-oxygen-requiring mode of energy production kicks in. Energy gets made, but at a cost: a buildup of lactic acid. The body's alkalinizing systems go on alert.

Maintenance of optimal good health hinges in part upon maintaining optimal pH in the body. The modern civilized human's diet works against this goal, because our favorite foods—meat, dairy, and grains—all have acidifying effects on the body. This does not mean that these foods are acidic in and of themselves; it means that when they are digested and assimilated, they cause acids to be produced within the body.

In many cases, unexplained low energy, aches, pains, or fatigue can be counteracted with an alkaline diet. Low-grade hyperacidity depletes energy and interferes with good digestion.

Take, for example, the case of Julie Billington's husband. He had been taking 10 to 12 Tums each day and continuing to complain of digestive problems and an acidic taste in his mouth. After a few days of using a green juice powder supplement, the problem reversed itself completely. Two years later, her husband hasn't had to use any antacids, and uses green juice daily instead. The benefit to Julie—aside from having a more healthy husband— is that the constant complaining has stopped!

Grains—even whole grains and sprouted grains—are acid-forming when digested. Sugars are extremely acid-forming. Meat and dairy are the most acid-forming foods you can eat. Green foods, on the other hand, are strongly alkaline.

This does not mean that eating too much bread or cheese will send you into a coma or respiratory arrest as soon as you finish that last bite. We're talking about extremely subtle alterations in pH, within narrow limits. Mainstream medicine, in its tradition of sailing in with heroic measures once disease is advanced, does not recognize these subtle fluctuations in pH as risk factors for any kind of disease. But natural medicine's case in favor of alkalinizing the body with plenty of green food—the most alkaline food you can consume—is growing.

When we eat a lot of acidifying food, our bodies have the ability to maintain proper alkalinity by freeing up minerals from the tissues. Potassium, magnesium, calcium, and other minerals are pulled from bones and other tissues to buffer excess acid. This can contribute to depletion of trace minerals— which, as you'll see in a later section, can have a significant impact on overall health. Short-term defense leads to long-term disease.

An over-acidic mouth can result when trace minerals are pulled from those tissues to maintain proper alkalinity. An alkaline diet aids in resistance against cavities, plaque, bleeding gums, periodontal disease and bad breath. Acidic pH in the mouth also affects our ability to enjoy the tastes of natural, raw, healthful foods, and we turn to sugar and fat to try to get that pleasurable taste-bud stimulation we feel we're missing.

Next time you crave sugar, swish some green juice in your mouth. As your mouth is alkalinized, your taste buds will come back to a more natural state, where they can experience the sweetness of a piece of fruit or a fresh vegetable.

Acidic environments in the body provide a less hostile environment for harmful bacteria, yeasts, and fungi (all of these can be described as pathogens) that can take a toll on human health. So, too, do low oxygen concentrations in parts of the physiology that are designed to be bathed in oxygen-rich blood as it circulates. The oxygenating power of chlorophyll and other components of green food, along with their alkalinizing properties, help to keep these putrefactive bacteria and other pathogens at bay. Improved oxygenation and alkalizing create an environment that is inhospitable to pathogenic organisms.

Some experts believe that acidity exacerbates autoimmune conditions such as rheumatoid arthritis, which could help to explain why a diet rich in fresh green food can help to relieve symptoms of those conditions.

## ACIDITY AND CANCER GROWTH

Cells within solid tumors are known to be more acidic than cells within normal tissues. It is accepted in oncological research that mechanisms that maintain intracellular pH at a more acidic level within cancer cells may be pivotal in preserving those cells and allowing them to multiply and spread. One of the most powerful ways to interrupt the incubation of carcinogenic substances is by alkalizing.

The results of several test-tube studies performed in cancer research laboratories in Canada and elsewhere have shown that manipulating cancer cells to alter their pH could be developed into a viable therapy for cancer in humans.

When we step back from the test tubes and microscopic experiments with cancerous cells and look at the incidence of cancer in various populations, it's easy to make a connection between an alkaline diet and cancer risk. Diets high in vegetables and fruit are clearly the best preventive medicine available against most cancers. Is this because of their alkalinizing effects, or due to their vitamin mineral content, or their antioxidant power? Most likely, it's an interactive picture, but it's a clear one: The more fresh, green food, the better.

## LACK OF ENZYMES IN THE DIET

An enzyme is a substance that is built from proteins, but it is so much more than a protein. Proteins aren't "alive" in the way enzymes are.

It appears that we inherit a certain enzyme-making potential at birth. We can deplete those enzymes quickly by sustaining ourselves on diets of cooked and processed foods—which are devoid of enzymes—or we can spare our bodies this rapid depletion by eating foods that are naturally rich in living enzymes: raw, fresh vegetables, fruits, and juices.

Some believe heating food at temperatures above 118 degrees Fahrenheit will denature (kill) all of its enzymes. This is not entirely true. Enzymes like Protease Lipase Cellulase and others do begin to be destroyed at that temperature theoretically, in reality however, many and most enzymes that we covet, the Super Oxide Dismutase, transhydrogenase fatty acid oxidase, peroxidase and others, can survive much higher temperatures. The real issue is what happens to proteins, fats, and carbohydrates when THEY are heated. Long before SOD is destroyed, proteins coagulate, fats degrade, volatile oils become deadly transfats, carbohydrates become cancer causing acrylamide and the life force is gone! Ditto for pasteurization, canning, and microwaving. Processing and cooking may make food safer in terms of its levels of harmful bacteria, but it makes it less safe by depleting the overall quality of our food.

If we don't get adequate enzymes through our diet, the digestive tract has fail-safe measures in place to obtain more enzyme power: It "robs" other parts of the body. After all, it's crucial for survival in the short-term to be able to break down food into its component nutrients. But over years and years of this kind of enzyme shuffling, some of the body's tissues become depleted. They age more rapidly and become more prone to degenerative, chronic conditions. One of the first places this is often seen is in the mouth and along the gums. Rinsing the mouth with fresh green juice—which is teeming with enzymes—is a helpful remedy for gingivitis and similar conditions that may be caused by enzyme depletion.

Wild cats and dogs eat raw meat and other fresh foods that are loaded with enzymes. Tests have shown that they have little to no enzyme activity in their saliva. Their domesticated counterparts, fed mostly high-carbohydrate, highly processed pet food, have a much higher salivary enzyme content. This is strong evidence that their enzyme production has been forced higher to assimilate these processed foods.

Decreased body enzyme levels occur in several chronic disease states, including allergies, skin diseases, cancer, and diabetes. Some animal research has linked diets deficient in enzymes to the premature onset of sexual maturity. Girls aged 8 or 9 today look a lot like girls of 12 or 13 looked 30 or so years ago. Some experts link this accelerated maturation to cooked- and processed-food diets—which tend to be higher in calories, speeding growth and sexual maturation—and to estrogen-mimicking chemical additives, which are believed to contribute to early onset of puberty.

Humans aren't made to eat processed, "dead" food, and neither are their pets. The prevalence of these foods in the bowls of the majority of domesticated animals may help to explain why cancer, heart disease, and other chronic ailments have become so common in house pets.

Think of an enzyme as a protein molecule with a potent "charge," like a battery. Enzyme researcher Edward Howell describes them as "the 'labor force' that builds your body, just like construction workers are the labor force that builds your house."

Enzymes are often referred to as 'catalysts' of biochemical reactions. Without those catalysts, all physiological function stops. If you don't have construction workers to nail the boards together to frame the house, those boards, nails, and hammers aren't of any use.

Over 2,000 distinct enzymes have been isolated and studied. For the most part, every enzyme has a specific function, serving as a particular "key" that will only lock into one particular *substrate* to "unlock" a single type of biochemical reaction.

I like to think of five distinct categories of enzymes, each with its own relationship to health and disease:

- *Metabolic enzymes*, which drive the processes of cellular repair, and the day-to-day work of transforming carbohydrates and fats into energy within individual cells;

- *Detoxification enzymes*, which work in the liver and elsewhere to transform toxins and carcinogenic substances, including drugs, into neutralized shadows of their former, toxic selves;[1]

---

1 *These enzymes are not all interchangeable. Each has its own specific role in the body. Metabolic enzymes can't do the work of detox enzymes, and detoxification enzymes can't do the work of antioxidant enzymes, and so on. On the other hand, the digestive enzymes, the antioxidant enzymes, and the enzymes found in raw*

- *Digestive enzymes,* made by the salivary glands, the stomach lining, and the pancreas, which work to break the foods we eat into their energy-producing basic components: carbohydrates, protein, and fat;

- *Enzymes found in raw foods,* which provide a natural complement to the digestive enzymes, promoting better digestion and reducing the need for pancreatic, salivary, and stomach-produced enzymes; and,

- *Enzymes found in food and produced in the body that have antioxidant power,* including glutathione peroxidase, catalase, and superoxide dismutase (SOD), a zinc- and copper-containing enzyme that is one of the body's most important defenses against the harmful effects of oxidation; these enzymes have their origin in the earliest time of plant evolution, when plants had to develop a number of antioxidant protection systems to prevent sun-induced oxidative damage; these enzymes are made in the body, but with aging, production falls, and increasing intake of antioxidants through (fresh, green) food is a sensible countermeasure.

Some of the most health-promoting nutrients found in green foods ascribe their health benefits, at least in part, to their effects on liver detoxification enzymes. For example: The nutrient *isothiocyanate sulforaphane,* found abundantly in broccoli, potently increases the activity of Phase II detoxification enzymes in the liver. (More on this in Chapter Six.)

## LACK OF TRACE MINERALS IN THE DIET

For too long it has been an accepted practice to supplement the diet with high doses of calcium. This is supposed to help prevent osteoporosis. But a close look at the research into calcium supplementation for osteoporosis prevention doesn't seem all that positive.

In the May 2005 issue of the medical journal *Lancet,* British researchers reported the results of a several-year study involving prevention of hip frac-

---

*foods can be functionally inter-changeable, with those found in foods supplementing those made by the body and doing the same jobs.*

tures with calcium and vitamin D. They enrolled just under 5,300 people aged 70 and up who had experienced a mild bone fracture and gave them either 1,000 mg of calcium a day, 800 IU of vitamin $D_3$ a day, or both. Some subjects got placebo pills. In the end, no combination of these supplements improved the subjects' chances of avoiding a second fracture.

Another study—this one in the *British Medical Journal*—looked at the effectiveness of calcium and vitamin $D_3$ (also known as cholecalciferol) for primary prevention of osteoporosis-related fractures. Over the 25-month follow-up period, the researchers did not detect any improvement in quality of life or decreased risk of fracture in the subjects on calcium, vitamin D, or a combination.

Here's the point: The body does not have the ability to absorb and utilize minerals in high doses, and if the human body simply can't absorb and utilize minerals in high doses, it cannot improve bone health or other parameters of wellness. Our intestines are made to absorb minerals and vitamins in trace amounts, in combination with one another—not in high doses in isolation.

Trace minerals—including selenium, fluoride, iron, zinc, iodine, copper, chromium, manganese, molybdenum, calcium, and magnesium—are found in our bodies in trace amounts. That's all we need. If we're going to use a mineral supplement to cover our bases, it's best to use one that gives us those minerals in trace amounts, in forms that are highly bioavailable.

Here's another example of poorly designed mineral supplementation: adding an iron supplement to the diet of a woman who thinks she's losing excess iron through menstruation. It is common practice to give a woman iron supplements without actually testing her for anemia. Iron can accumulate in her body, promoting toxicity and excessive oxidation, (aging!)

Women commonly are advised to take iron during pregnancy, too, but this can have adverse effects. Some experts have hypothesized that slight anemia during pregnancy has advantages for fetal survival. And iron tablets are one of the most common causes of toddler poisoning deaths.

A well-designed trace mineral supplement, like Ionic Elements, contains a balanced amount of the various minerals required by the body. It complements and mimics the natural mineral content of the most nutritious foods—those that are deep green in color. Any deficiencies can be remedied with this approach. Mineral megadoses simply aren't necessary.

## DIFFICULT OR STAGNANT ELIMINATIVE FUNCTION

You've probably heard it said that death begins in the colon. This phrase is just a little more colorful than it needs to be, but it does hold a kernel of truth.

Ancient Egyptian physicians were the first to describe a condition called *autointoxication*, where wastes would get backed up in the large intestine because of poor elimination. Toxins in that waste would then be absorbed back into the circulation through the intestinal walls to wreak continued havoc throughout the body. The ancient Greeks called it *putrefaction*.

Elie Metchnikoff, the Russian scientist who first described the salutary effects of probiotic bacteria on human health, also pointed out that toxins in the large intestine can shorten human life span if they aren't either expelled or neutralized. The basic concept remained, despite the various names it was given; we become poisoned by our own waste if it isn't eliminated in a timely fashion.

Inflammatory bowel disease, characterized by pain and diarrhea, is believed to be caused by bacterial overgrowth. When waste sits too long in the GI tract, the chances increase that harmful bacteria will take root, reproduce, and cause problems.

There are commonalities between the old concept of autointoxication and a relatively new—and increasingly common—condition known as *multiple chemical sensitivity* (MCS). The symptom profiles of the two are strikingly similar. Some experts believe that the two are one and the same.

Chronic constipation is a known risk factor for cancer of the colon. In one large study, it was found that frequent constipation—serious enough for the subject to want to take a laxative to treat it, on more than 52 days of the year, for a period of 10 years—increased risk of colon cancer by almost four-and-a-half times. Another study found that three or fewer bowel movements per week increased colon cancer risk twofold.

Green, fresh food is by far the best remedy for sluggish elimination. Second best would be fiber both soluble and dietary like that found in seeds, nuts, grains, beans, and legumes. Stimulant laxatives, even natural versions, can be addicting, creating a situation where the user needs laxatives to have normal bowel function.

The living enzymes in fresh, raw food help to ensure that meals are thoroughly broken down before they get to the large intestine. Low enzymes can leave some food unprocessed, and when it hits the colon, bacteria start to finish the job, producing gas and cramping and increasing the likelihood of constipation.

If you don't believe me, just try this: Eat nothing but fresh, raw green food and fruit for a day, and be sure to drink plenty of water. See how things go the next morning. If you add fresh grass juice or vegetable juices, the results will likely provide further validation of the value of green foods for gastrointestinal "regularity."

## FERMENTED (CULTURED) PLANT FOODS

Fermented foods have been a staple of the human diet for thousands of years. Fermentation, also known as culturing, was originally developed as a method of food preservation. Cultured foods are alive with micro-organisms and enzymes, help regulate the level of acidity in the digestive tract, and contain multiple compounds that act as antioxidants. Many of these foods are rich in isothiocyanates, which help prevent cancer.

Fermentation is an anaerobic process, which means that it takes place in the absence of oxygen. Friendly bacteria (including *Lactobacillus* and *Bifidum* bacteria), yeasts (usually, *S. boulardii*), or molds are used to break down carbohydrates, in essence "pre-digesting" the food and altering it in health-promoting ways. The friendly "bugs" used for fermentation aid the digestive system by allowing beneficial microflora to colonize in the intestines. A fermented food is, essentially, a raw food, alive with energy—as long as it has not been pasteurized. Fermentation also produces beneficial enzymes and allows the body to absorb vitamins and minerals more effectively.

Probiotics are particularly important when taking antibiotics, since antibiotics kill off all bacteria—the bad and the good. Other drugs, excess alcohol, stress, disease, toxic exposure, or even antibacterial soap can all reduce the body's levels of digestive bacteria. By strengthening digestive flora with regular consumption of cultured plant foods, you will strengthen your immunity and make your body less vulnerable to infection.

It is important that you try to find raw (unpasteurized) fermented vegetables that contain active or live cultures. Pasteurizing kills the living bacteria, making it less beneficial than its non-pasteurized counterpart.

Cucumbers, beets, turnips, green tomatoes, peppers, lettuces, cabbage, eggplant, onion, squash, and carrots are all used across the globe for lacto-fermentation. Miso, a fermented soybean paste, is a flavorful, salty ingredient used often in Japanese cuisine. Kimchi, also called gimchi or kimchee, is a traditional fermented Korean dish consisting of vegetables—usually Chinese cabbage—and chili peppers. Scientists have found that Kimchi can be used to treat avian influenza, otherwise known as bird flu. Sauerkraut, which is fermented cabbage, offers an excellent source of vitamin C, lactobacilli, and other nutrients.

## TOXIC EXPOSURES

The role of exposure to chemical toxins in our declining levels of wellness is only beginning to be recognized as such by the medical main-stream, but alternative medicine has acknowledged its importance for decades.

According to a fact sheet published by the National Institutes of Health, there are approximately 15,000 chemicals currently in high-volume use in the United States. America's production of various chemicals tops 300 billion pounds per year. These chemicals are used to make building materials for our homes and offices, to aid in the growth of crops, to make fabrics and soaps and solvents, and hundreds of other uses.

Many thousands of other chemicals are unintentionally created as by-products of industry, such as the methylmercury that has been found in the flesh of virtually every kind of fish, and the dioxins that appear to be more and more common in the tissues of humans and the breast milk of nursing mothers.

Some chemicals are life-saving and necessary. Some chemicals play important roles in manufacturing or the production of energy. But many are toxic to the human body, harming our reproductive health, predisposing us to cancer, or causing us to "react" with allergy, mysterious fatigue, pain, or other symptoms. Many collect in our tissues as we consume foods that contain them.

The research on this subject is still young, but one thing is clear: Green foods have powerful detoxifying effects against some of these chemicals. Chlorella, which will be discussed in greater detail in Chapter Five, and the fresh juice of cereal grasses, discussed in Chapter Four, are especially cleansing.

## LIVING GREEN, BEATS DYING!

In the beginning, Reba had decided that she wasn't going to drink what she called "the nasty green stuff." She knew it was good for her, but couldn't go to the next level of actually trying it.

One day she felt headachy and low. On a whim, she decided she'd go ahead and try that green stuff after all. Twenty minutes later, she felt incredible. The headache was gone.

A few days later, she felt the beginnings of a migraine. If you've ever had one of these headaches, you know that they can be knock-you-out awful, and that they don't go away by themselves. She mixed a soup spoon-sized serving of greens powder into a glass of juice and drank it down. The migraine was gone in a matter of minutes.

Reba is now drinking her "nasty green stuff " every day, and loving it.

Addressing chronic disease by eating more vegetables and fruits in their raw state—and, if you choose, adding green supplements to your diet—isn't any guarantee that you will remain hearty. It will, however, vastly improve your quality of life and energy levels the very day you start your program.

Within weeks, a diet rich in vegetables, fruit, and concentrated green "su-perfoods" will reduce inflammation, improve elimination, and reduce oxidation's toll on your body. Some green foods will speed the elimination of toxins from your body and protect you against the DNA damage and oxidation they can foster. They'll boost your intake of enzymes and alkalinize your body. You will lose weight, which will in turn reduce your risk of many chronic diseases. It's worth sacrificing the junk food and the sugar to have all this, right?

If not, consider this: Every time you do have a little something that is on the not-so-good side, be thankful that green foods will be there to balance the scales and clean-up the mess.

# Chapter Four

## CEREAL GRASSES

Grains as highly processed flour, often with added sugars, and calling it food is pretty terrible for your health. Too many refined grains lead to rapid and dramatic fluctuations in blood sugar, which then lead to further cravings for refined grains and their more lethal cousin, refined sugars. Diets high in refined grains and sugars set you up for type 2 diabetes, obesity, food allergy, and heart disease. They encourage the growth of harmful *Candida* yeasts in the GI tract, sinuses, and genitourinary tract. Some research suggests that they also predispose us to chronic inflammation and even cancer. These processed grains have been stripped of all the nutritional gifts of whole grain, compounding the liabilities of a diet high in these foods by essentially depleting your body of needed vitamins and minerals.

On the other hand, the cultivation of grains has been a major factor in enabling the earth's resources to feed so many billions of people. Grains are calorically dense and easily stored. Seems like a bit of a catch-22: Although refined grains are not the best food for our health, they feed large numbers of mouths each day that might not otherwise be fed.

The fabulous thing about grains is not that they can be husked and pulverized to make flour. It's that they are *seeds*. Seeds that, if grown properly, will yield brilliant green shoots of grass, infused with life energy and packed with life-giving nutrients: vitamins, minerals, chlorophyll, and enzymes.

Seeds are amazing. Remember when, as a child, you first realized that an acorn was all it took to make that gigantic oak tree in your front yard? Remember when you realized that planting a tiny seed and giving it some water and sun could yield a bumper crop of tomatoes, or zucchini, or sugar snap peas? We've lost that sense of wonder in a sea of snack cakes and sliced white bread that resembles styrofoam more than it resembles anything from nature. That white bread acts like glue in your gut. Not a pretty picture.

It's time to put our grains to better use by sprouting them and partaking of the green stuff that springs from them. This step alone can make a huge difference in your health—and can give you an energy boost that must be experienced to be appreciated.

Incidentally, whole grains are healthful foods that could be a part of a super foods lifestyle. Brown and germinated barley, oats, and quinoa are all delicious, hearty additions to a plant-based diet.

Here's another reason to consume the green sprouts from grains in addition to the grain itself: A blade of wheatgrass is far more nutrient-dense, calorie for calorie, than the grain of wheat from which it sprouts. We Westerners are not lacking on the calorie front—in fact, most of us eat a few hundred more calories per day than we require. Even if we don't pack on the pounds from this regular overconsumption of calories, our bodies still have to go through the labor of **processing** all of those calories. This takes a toll. It ages us more rapidly and depletes our energy and life force.

While individuals may be allergic to grains, have gastrointestinal discomforts when they eat grains, or have full-blown celiac disease (gluten intolerance), the grasses that sprout from grains are non-allergenic. It's estimated that a million Americans have undiagnosed celiac disease—where their bodies can't properly digest gluten, the main protein in wheat, barley, oats, and other grains. It is estimated that only *3 percent* of people with celiac disease have been properly diagnosed. If you have chronic gastrointestinal discomfort—sometimes diagnosed as irritable bowel syndrome—or chronic allergies, eczema, or asthma, try eliminating all gluten-containing grains for two weeks (that's basically all grains besides rice and corn). I bet you'll be astonished at how much you improve. You can continue to use fresh wheat or barley grass juices while on a gluten-free diet.

There are several varieties of grasses from grains—which are generally referred to as *cereal grasses*—that you can choose from. In my teachings, I recommend several varieties, including barley grass and a special form of wheatgrass, Green Kamut, which I'll tell you more about later in this chapter.

## THE FRESH GRASS JUICE EXPERIENCE

If you haven't done so already, it's time for you to step into a juice bar or health food shop and have a shot of wheatgrass juice.

Before you drink it down, take a good look at it. You've probably never seen anything of this exact shade of emerald green. Take a sniff; it smells like a mowed lawn on a spring day, but sweeter, and without the herbicides! Then, a small sip. The taste might take some getting used to; it's not a bad taste, but it's definitely...grassy.

Toss the rest of the shot into your mouth and swish it around. It might make your mouth tingle. Then, swallow it. Don't forget to thank your friendly juice bar/health-food store employee for that shot of liquid sunshine.

Pay attention to how you are feeling over the next few minutes. If you didn't have that wheatgrass on top of a heavy meal, you will soon begin to feel a surge of energy and a sense of improved clarity. It's nothing like the feeling you get from coffee or a concentrated dose of sugar; it's a steady, focused, even *blissful* kind of energy. This is the grass juice experience, and in the rest of this chapter I'm going to tell you why grass juices make you feel so good today—and why, if you make them a regular part of your life, they can make a big difference in your long-term state of health.

Wheatgrass, Kamut grass, and barley grass juices can do much more than keep you healthy. I've seen what I'd call miraculous turnarounds in the waning health of very sick people, on regimens that hinge upon regular consumption of concentrated cereal grasses.

Sandra had been suffering from ulcerative colitis for years. She had been taking steroid medications to treat the colitis for a year; these drugs had caused her to feel weak and short-tempered, and had caused her to gain weight (all common side effects in people who use these medications). Eventually, she tired of the side effects and stopped using the drugs. She began to look for other solutions. When she began to consume wheatgrass juice daily—along with a primarily raw and overall very healthful diet—her stools became normal; her abdominal pain ceased; and she had a huge increase in energy.

Ulcerative colitis is a disorder that is considered chronic and incurable, but Sandra was able to heal herself naturally—a huge achievement that saved her a lifelong battle with steroid side effects.

Another wheatgrass convert, Ellen, started out with hypoglycemia (blood sugar that dips too low soon after a meal, leading to shakiness, clouded thinking, and intense cravings for refined carbohydrates), chronic yeast infections, headaches, bloating, flatulence, and constipation. She entered the raw foods program at Hippocrates, which gave her a jump-start on a raw foods program that included plenty of wheatgrass juice. Her symptoms disappeared rapidly, and she reported clearer thinking and abundant energy that allowed her to accomplish more every day.

Asthma is another chronic condition that has physicians stumped. It can be treated with drugs, but those drugs often make the problem worse in the long run; studies show that overuse of fast-acting inhalers that relieve shortness of breath can end up causing attacks, and increase the likelihood of dying from the disease. Increasing numbers of children are being diagnosed with this disease, and believe themselves doomed to a lifetime of medicines to keep their airways open. George, another graduate of the Hippocrates Health Institute's program, noticed immediate improvement in his asthma after only a few days on the raw foods program. And he lost around eight pounds while on that program! Another asthma patient, Ginny, had been on asthma drugs every day since she was a small child. She told me that transitioning to wheatgrass and living food had cured her completely.

Cancer patients have also reported seemingly miraculous cures with the Hippocrates program, including lots of grass juices. Simon was diagnosed with cancer of the colon that had metastasized (spread) far enough that removal of the entire colon was recommended. He refused the surgery—a mark of enormous courage!—and entered into the raw foods and wheat-grass juicing program. His pain, which had been intense, faded over the course of a few months, and the cancer actually disappeared, according to the results of tests he had just before writing about his experience.

Cereal grass juices are most effective at healing or preventing disease when they are used in concert with the raw foods diet. The Hippocrates program is quite intensive, and if you are seriously ill or seriously motivated to prevent illness, you may want to investigate participating in it or a program like it. But if you are not prepared to go to the extreme of stopping your life and going off for a while to cleanse, purify, and heal, you can still take the proactive step of adding cereal grass juices to your life. You can do this today, without changing anything else, and you will benefit greatly.

You'll learn in this chapter how to choose the best source of grass power for your needs.

## WHEATGRASS JUICE: WHAT IS IT?

Wheatgrass is the green, growing plant that will eventually become a shaft of wheat, which will then produce seeds (grain), die, and be harvested. Those seeds are a major staple of the standard modern diet. But the wheat-grass plant is another thing altogether.

While grains are an overused food staple in many developed parts of the world—particularly grains that have been highly refined and ground into flour—the green plant that is the beginnings of those grains is purely and simply a vegetable. Within only seven days of being cultivated, a tray of wheatgrass plants can reach six to nine inches in height, and at that point they can be cut and juiced; or they can be chewed as they are—juiced in the mouth and the fibrous parts spit out.

Cereal grass juices are available in other forms too. Health food retailers may carry various brands of powdered grass juices that are easier to use on a day-to-day basis. Some of these powders maintain much of the vitality of the original juices because of careful processing; others don't.

Wheatgrass juice is abundant with vitamins, minerals, enzymes, and chlorophyll. When you drink a shot of fresh wheatgrass juice, you also imbibe the plant's vital life energy—energy that is tapped at the exact point in the plant's growth where its life energy is at its peak.

If grass is so great, why aren't people going out into green pastures and grazing like cattle? Because growing grass for human consumption as a health food is a bit more involved than munching on whatever's springing up from the soil in your backyard.

## CEREAL GRASSES: THEIR HISTORY ON THE PLANET

In the late Cenozoic period—10 to 15 million years before the writing of this book—grasses became a major part of the earth's ecosystem. The spread of grasses across the globe led to a dramatic rise in the populations of ruminant animals: the predecessors of today's cows, oxen, sheep, goats, and deer. Ruminants are the owners of four distinct stomachs, which enable them to thoroughly digest the grasses they subsist on in the wild.

Today, there are about 9,000 species of grasses on earth. They grow preferentially in areas of low rainfall, such as the North American plains, South American savannahs, and the African veldt.

Grasses use a slightly different form of photosynthesis than do shrubs and trees. This process helped them to thrive when atmospheric carbon dioxide levels were low and the earth's temperatures were cooler. Today, as $CO_2$ levels rise and temperatures go up along with them, grasses aren't finding the planet to be quite as hospitable as they once did.

Species of the grass family are enormously important to humans, providing the base of the food chain. Not only do grasses feed the animals we like to eat, but they also yield the grains—wheat, barley, rye, millet, corn, oats, rice—that made civilization possible, and that today yield the lion's share of the calories eaten on the planet. In the year 2001 alone, a total of 567.3 million tons of wheat were grown worldwide.

Most animals raised for food also eat grains, in addition to hay, which is made from dried grass, sorghum, timothy, and fescue. Sugarcane and sorghum, both grasses, are used to make sugar and molasses, and even provide raw materials for the making of corn starch and paper. Bamboo, another type of grass, is used for construction. Grasses have large root systems that make them perfect allies in erosion control.

Grasses, along with lilies, orchids, and palms, belong to the plant family of *monocotyledons*. They send up a single seed-leaf, have straight veins, and have flowers that form in multiples of three. They can be munched down to the ground and grow back, providing a reliable source of food for the world's grazing animals.

Anyone who has marveled at the way stems of grass can emerge through sidewalks, streets, walls, and rocks knows how hardy this plant family is. Grasses have been around a long time. This plant family has successfully run the gauntlet of natural selection; over millions of years of "survival of the fittest," grass has shown itself to be uniquely adapted to life on this planet. Not coincidentally, grasses are also perfectly suited to be a food source for the creatures that evolved after it—not only the ruminants, but the humans as well.

We don't have the stomach power to digest grass whole, but we do have the big brains necessary to figure out how to extract the nutrients in grass and use them to our benefit.

Enter Charles Schnabel and his ailing hens.

## PIONEERING RESEARCH INTO CEREAL GRASSES: DR. CHARLES SCHNABEL

In 1930, agricultural chemist Charles Schnabel's chickens fell ill. When he fed them young, tender grass, an amazing healing response was elicited, and an increase in fertility to boot.

During the course of this experiment, Dr. Schnabel had noticed that the chickens preferred the younger grass to older shoots. This curious scientist set out to discover what was so special about the grass on which his chickens had thrived, and ended up devoting much of his professional life to the study of grass.

In an article published in 1973 in the journal *Acres, USA*, Schnabel wrote that "the average person needs 205 pounds of 'leafy, green and yellow' vegetables a year, but receipt records indicate that approximately one bushel (about 20 pounds) of fresh greens per capita were used annually in eight large cities before World War II...Apparently, then, the average city dweller eats less than one-fourth as much greens as he should. Is it any wonder that we suffer from colds, are perpetually tired and develop degenerative diseases before we reach the age when we should be in the prime of life?"

Dr. Schnabel's words, though written several decades before the turn of the twenty-first century, could well make reference to today's city dwellers, and most country and suburban dwellers, too. Most of us still haven't caught on to the enormous importance of fresh green food in our diets—and the difference it would make in the nation's health if every person got seven to nine servings of vegetables and fruit each day.

Dr. Schnabel's research yielded important insights into the growth pattern of cereal grasses—finding out why his chickens preferred grass at a particular stage of growth, the *jointing* stage. (Jointing is sometimes referred to as segmentation.) Again, from the article, a passage both informative and poetic:

*"Since grazing animals are parasites on plants the different plant families have adopted characteristic methods of protecting themselves from destruction. The trees hold their leaves out of reach. The cactus developed spines. Many plants develop poisons in their leaves... But the grasses solved this problem of self-preservation in a way far different from any other plant family. They joint. All grasses, at maturity, like the bamboo fishing pole, have numerous joints or nodes—but it is the formation of the first joint that holds the age-old secret of grass...*

*If the grass culm is cut or grazed before the first joint forms it will grow up again, but if cut after that time it will die. This fact has been known for centuries but no significance has been attached to it since 1931, when it was discovered that all grass leaves reach a peak of food value, per pound of dry matter, on the day the first joint begins to form...this simple discovery may well change the course of history because it taps the cheapest and best source of vitamins in the world."*

He found that "grazing animals never eat *jointed* grass if there is any unjointed grass available," and that grass was highest in nutritional value at the very end of the stage of unjointed growth, and that if it was allowed to continue to grow into the jointed stage, much of that nutrition would be lost.

Unjointed grass does not have a stem, as more mature grass plants do. Grass planted in fertile soils will joint within three weeks of planting as long as the weather is warm and they get enough water. Left to grow unfettered, the jointed grass will then yield mature grain in about 80 days' time. But if they are cut just before jointing, they make what by nutritional measures is just about a nearly perfect food.

The grasses are unique in the plant world because of this huge marshalling of energy and resources to prepare for the big growth spurt that occurs during jointing. If we snip and juice the grass just at that point before it joints, we not only preserve the plant's root so that it can send up another shoot, we also catch that perfect green food at its pinnacle of nutritional value.

In one study, Dr. Schnabel fed guinea pigs diets of single foods: cabbage, carrots, head lettuce, canned spinach, or dried grass powder; some animals got a mixed diet of all the vegetables besides grass. The growth curves of each animal were recorded and put onto graphs.

The difference in the growth of grass-fed animals and those on the other diets was enormous. And when animals fed the other foods were shifted to the grass diet, their growth curves shot upward. He also mentions a farm where the egg-producing life spans of hens were quadrupled when grasses were added to their diets of alfalfa. Further studies found that cows fed dehydrated grass juice had significant increases in milk production. (Dr. Schnabel found no difference in effectiveness or nutrient content between gently dehydrated grass juice and fresh. Keep this in mind, because it can make a big difference in the accessibility of these foods in your busy life.)

"Only one-half ounce of 40 percent protein dehydrated grass would supply 18,600 units of vitamin A [as beta-carotene], 113 milligrams of vitamin C, and 5 to 7 grams of the best quality protein in the world. This is more vitamin A than is supplied by the entire 84.5 ounces of food in the optimum diet, and more vitamin C than is supplied by the entire 30 ounces of fruits and vegetables...there is no other total solution to the human nutrition problem. Even if vitamins A and C could be synthesized to retail at their yardstick values this would not supply all the other vitamins which are associated with vitamins A and C."

Dr. Schnabel was on to something. Current research has built on the foundation he laid with his research on chickens, guinea pigs, and dairy cows. He had found a way to tap into the nutritional bounty of grasses without four stomachs—and he believed that doing so would be a crucial part of adequately nourishing the world's population in the years to come.

Most of the world still hasn't caught on, but I hope to help change that.

## CEREAL GRASSES' NUTRIENT CONTENT

Wheat isn't the only grain from which intensely green juices can be harvested before segmentation. Wheatgrass is more readily available in its fresh form, but other cereal grasses—notably, barley and Kamut grasses— have their own advantages.

Barley and wheatgrass are roughly equal in nutrient density. Their chlorophyll content is the same, and their therapeutic value is about equal, too. Barley and wheatgrasses can be used to aid healing from the same spectrum of disorders. All cereal grasses vary in nutrient density according to the richness of the soil in which they are grown, and the overall growing conditions. Although the grains (seeds) of both plants contain the protein *gluten*, to which many people are allergic, the grasses from which they grow contain no gluten at all. Even people with celiac disease—characterized by diarrhea and pain any time gluten is consumed—can supplement their diets safely with cereal grasses.

Kamut is a strain of wheat that is believed to have originated in the cradle of civilization—the Nile area of Egypt—and it is one of the most ancient members of the wheat family. Its cultivation is believed to have begun over 4,000 years ago.

## THE SOLDIER AND THE STOLEN GRAIN

Legend has it that Kamut arrived in North America after the Second World War. It's said that an American pilot found some of this grain preserved in a stone box in an Egyptian tomb. The kernels found their way to a Montana wheat farmer, who planted them and brought the resulting harvest to a local fair, where they earned the nickname "King Tut's Wheat."

After that, the legend goes, the grain was not grown again in North America until the late 1970s, when another Montana wheat farmer got hold of a jar of King Tut's Wheat and put considerable effort into propagating this unique, sweet form of hard amber spring wheat. This enterprising farmer,

T. Mack Quinn, dubbed it Kamut—the ancient Egyptian word for wheat. Quinn's family registered Kamut as a trademark. Since that time, its popularity has grown, and it has proven hardy enough to grow well under organic growing conditions.

Source: Quinn, Robert M., "Kamut®: Ancient Grain, New Cereal," *Perspectives on New Crops and New Uses*, ASHS Press, Alexandria, VA; posted at http://www.hort.purdue.edu/newcrop/proceedings1999/v4-182.html

In its whole-grain, seed form, Kamut has a nutty, almost buttery flavor. It is used to make crackers and cereals, and contains less gluten—the allergenic protein that many people have problems tolerating—than other, more modern grains like durum wheat. Kamut is 20 to 40 percent higher in protein than durum wheat, and contains higher concentrations of essential fats, vitamins, and minerals as well. This higher concentration of nutrient power carries over into the tender green leaves that sprout from it. You can use those leaves to make an organic, non-hybridized wheatgrass called Green Kamut.

Green Kamut is a green juice made from organically grown Kamut leaves. These deep green leaves are a highly pure source of nutrient-rich food. They are 100 percent organic.

I have found a way that is capable of taking the young plants into nutrient- and enzyme-rich juice, and then into a powder extract, using a proprietary process that requires absolutely no binders or fillers.

A kernel of Kamut is two to three times larger than a kernel of wheat. The grain itself is believed to be less allergenic and more nutrient-dense than modern wheat, making it a healthful substitute for wheat in breads and cereals. It is higher in protein than conventional wheat.

Research into barley grass has focused on its detoxifying properties. wheatgrass has these properties as well.

Ann Wigmore:

*"The enzymes and amino acids found in wheatgrass can protect us from carcinogens like no other food or medicine can. It strengthens our cells, detoxifies the liver [and] bloodstream, and chemically neutralizes environmental pollutants...Recent studies show that wheatgrass juice has a powerful ability to fight tumors without the usual toxicity of drugs that also inhibit cell-destroying agents".*

—from *The Wheatgrass Book*

## JUICE FROM GRASS: HOW IT'S DONE

Wheatgrass can be grown outdoors, in fields, or indoors in trays. You can grow your own for juicing at home, and harvest it just before jointing in 9 to 12 days. Or, you can let someone else do the work for you and dehydrate the juice, drastically increasing the nutrient density of the green food that ends up in your body.

The basics on growing your own can be found on page **130.** If you are concerned that you might not be able to get the full benefit of cereal grass juice because of an unwillingness to turn your home into a grassy veldt, rest easy; dehydrated grass juices are actually more concentrated sources of nutrients than fresh. A fresh glass of wheatgrass juice is mostly water.

## WHEATGRASS AS A NATURAL THERAPY

Wheatgrass juice was one of Ann Wigmore's favorite all-purpose remedies for a wide variety of conditions. Its combination of nutrients, enzymes, and amino acids (protein building blocks) work to fill in deficiencies and activate the innate healing potential of each individual's body. For example:

- A small study involving 21 ulcerative colitis patients found that wheatgrass juice significantly reduced their symptoms.

- Dehydrated grass juices are permitted to carry a national Seal of Approval for use by diabetics. Grady Brown, a type 2 diabetic, credits wheatgrass for the reduction of his blood sugars from a steady 518-plus to a steady 85 to 110—well within normal levels. "All diabetics should take this!" he wrote in his testimonial.

- A wheatgrass enema has powerful detoxifying effects. Dr. Wigmore suggests holding the juice in the bowel for 20 minutes.

- Itchy skin is soothed almost immediately with topical application of wheatgrass juice; so, too, are cuts, scrapes, burns, poison ivy, insect bites, athlete's foot, boils, and sores. Sunburn, too, can be treated in this way. Alternatively, a poultice made from cut blades of young grass can be used for skin conditions.

- Gargling and rinsing the mouth with wheatgrass juice freshens breath and helps to reduce inflammation of the gums (gingivitis) and periodontitis. Research suggests that regularly rinsing the mouth with grass juice may help prevent the formation of mouth ulcers and oral cancers. The presence of a specific antioxidant enzyme called *superoxide dismutase*, or SOD, in wheatgrass—and in other cereal grasses—may help to explain some of these healing effects.

## CEREAL GRASS JUICES CONTAIN SUPEROXIDE DISMUTASE (SOD)

Several kinds of free radicals are formed in body cells as a normal part of metabolism, detoxification, and immune system function. One of the most potent and potentially harmful of these radicals is the superoxide radical, which is implied in the genesis of arthritis and cancer.

Many types of cancer cells have been found to be deficient in the enzyme that Nature designed to "quench" the superoxide radical: superoxide dismutase (SOD). Animal and human studies show that the joint tissues of osteoarthritis sufferers have lower concentrations of SOD. Superoxide radicals break down the components of synovial fluid, the viscous material that helps cushion the ends of bones as they move against one another. When patients with knee osteoarthritis received injections of SOD into the affected joint three times a day, their pain was reduced substantially, and they were able to walk normally and to climb stairs again.

At the cellular level, SOD has been found to protect cells against the biological transmutations that can turn them cancerous.

## CEREAL GRASS, DNA, AND CANCER

In the modern world, we are constantly bombarded with carcinogens and radiation from many sources. The body is under assault, and although we may not feel the cumulative effects of this day-to-day toxic warfare, it takes its toll on our bodies, a few cells at a time. Over the years, this could predispose us to developing any of a number of common chronic diseases—most notably (and frighteningly), one of dozens of forms of cancer.

Current statistics show that one of every two men is likely to have some form of cancer in his lifetime, and that women have only slightly better chances of escaping a cancer diagnosis: Their odds are one in three. Many experts are convinced that the cancer epidemic is directly attributable to a combination of two factors: 1) an overabundant yet nutrient-poor diet, and 2) day-to-day exposure to synthetic chemical toxins used in or created as wastes by industry, or those commonly found in building materials, new mattresses and carpets, plastics, paint, glue, solvents, car exhaust, incinerated waste, cleaning supplies, and even children's toys.

The second factor creates damage at the very heart of our cells: the DNA that codes for each healthy cell. The first factor deprives our bodies of its natural defenses against this damage.

The initial event of carcinogenesis is a change in cellular DNA that causes the cell to become *undifferentiated*—unable to do its unique job in the body.

These cells then cannot work as a part of a tissue or organ system, and instead they take up space, multiplying and growing. Cancer cells do not have the natural "clock" that causes healthy cells to eventually self- destruct, a phenomenon known as apoptosis. So, these cells that are not of any use to the body grow rapidly and use up the body's energy supply without doing any work.

According to current research, the concentrated nutrition found in cereal grasses could well repair that DNA damage before it gets out of hand. Studies on barley grass are especially promising.

Barley grass is taken from young barley plants. This superfood—along with wheatgrass—has been widely sold as a nutritional supplement since before World War II. Barley grass has been especially popular and intensively researched in Japan in recent decades.

Biologist Jasuo Hotta, working at the University of Southern California at La Jolla, set out to research the reparative effects of powdered barley grass juice on damaged DNA—the genetic material that creates the "blueprints" from which nearly all body cells are made. Damage to DNA by carcinogens is a major route through which chemical toxins push the shift of cells from healthy to cancerous, and Hotta's studies were based on a foundation of many others that had shown the promise of green food in repairing this kind of damage.

Dr. Hotta and co-workers added powdered barley grass to cells with damaged DNA. The DNA of those cells repaired itself at twice the speed of cells that were left to their own devices. In another experiment, they exposed cells isolated in a test-tube to a carcinogen and radiation at the same time. Barley grass juice was added to some of the cell cultures, and those cells repaired themselves at least three times faster than cells without the green juice.

## PHYSICIAN, DETOXIFY AND REJUVENATE—WITH GREEN FOOD

One best-selling author and anti-aging physician names green foods like barley grass and wheatgrass as number 6 on his list of 10 Superfoods. (He also includes blue-green algae, a class of foods that includes spirulina and chlorella.)

Dr. Howard Lutz, Director of the Institute of Preventive Medicine in Washington, D.C., had chronic fatigue for many years. After trying every natural therapy he could find—without success—he attended the Ann Wigmore Institute in Boston. He began to drink wheatgrass juice daily, and soon noticed a dramatic improvement in his energy level. For the first time in years, he was able to work at his job for 10 to 12 hours a day.

In a conversation with a radio listener—I didn't catch his name, so let's call him Bill—I was told that he had visited an M.D. who happened to be considering making an investment in a health food company. (Let's call him Dr. Jones.) Dr. Jones was skeptical, but Bill gave him a wakeup call by pointing out the doctor's creased earlobes—a known sign of increased risk of heart attack. In addition, Dr. Jones was overweight, tired-looking, and had unhealthy looking skin, and knew it. He told Bill that he'd love to try the Plant Based Nutrition Program I designed.

After three months on the program, Dr. Jones reported experiencing extra energy and stamina, along with a feeling of well-being that he had never experienced before. He was losing from one-and-a-half to two pounds each month. Dr. Jones told Bill that he felt that this was the only regimen that provides safe, effective, slow, and permanent weight reduction. He also mentioned that Mrs. Jones was happy to see him on a weight-loss program that didn't make him grumpy and difficult, as others had done.

Barley grass, wheatgrass, and Kamut all have similar healing properties. All of these juices have been used successfully by natural medicine to aid in healing from allergies, anemia, arthritis, asthma, chronic fatigue, constipation, skin injuries or infections by fungus or bacteria, and yeast infections.

This green juice also has detoxifying effects beyond its protection of DNA threatened by carcinogens or radiation; it also promotes the proper function of the natural detoxification systems within the liver that work constantly to neutralize and dispose of potentially toxic substances, including synthetic chemicals and heavy metals:

- Juice from unjointed grass is loaded with chlorophyll, which improves *intestinal motility*—the ability of the muscular intestinal wall to move waste out of the body through bowel movements. Most green juice converts who tend towards constipation notice quick relief from this problem, which is not only uncomfortable, but increases the likelihood that toxins in the bowel will be reabsorbed into the body (a process known as *entero-hepatic recirculation*). In many cases, reabsorbed toxins have been "activated" in the bowel by bacteria, making them even more toxic.

- Studies show that green grass juices and other green foods can decrease the absorption of toxic chemicals, such as dioxins, through the walls of the intestine into the body. It decreases the absorption of dioxins—and, possibly, other toxic chemicals—through the walls of the intestinal tract into the bloodstream. When animals are dosed with heavy metals (mercury, lead) or dioxins and given concentrated green food, the excretion of these poisons into their feces increases significantly over their less fortunate lab animal brethren.

- More research from our old friend Dr. Schnabel: Hens fed cereal grasses and then killed for the dinner table proved to have "dark mahogany" colored livers—an indicator of good liver health—while the hens who had been fed alfalfa had much paler, sickly looking livers.

## DEHYDRATED GRASSES

Cereal grass juices that are dehydrated at low temperatures can preserve all of the plant's nutrients and enzymes. If you choose a dehydrated cereal grass over fresh, ensure that it is processed at a low temperature (88 degrees Fahrenheit) and not pasteurized, and that it is processed within a few hours of being cut. Dehydrated wheat and barley grass juices are good choices, and can be complemented with the juice of Kamut leaves. All these plants are slightly different in their nutritional composition. Find the ones that work best for you. By refreshing your cells with a variety of green foods, you can go for a lifetime without ever diminishing.

One young man, Matt Goodman, was diagnosed with multiple sclerosis just shy of his 26th birthday, with intense fatigue, numbness in his arms and legs, tremors, vertigo, incontinence, and vision problems. Two years later, he began to educate himself about natural healing methods, reading extensively and studying with renowned healers. He experimented with supplements and foods with special healing benefits. Matt soon began to recognize that MS hadn't attacked him out of the blue, but that it was his body's reaction to foods and lifestyle that went against the natural order of things. Fasting, yoga, meditation, raw foods, and massage were all aspects of his plan for moving back in the direction of health. He also used products I designed, including Green Kamut, Spirulina, and Activated Barley.

In 2003, Matt and his dog Jerry completed a 1,600-mile hike along the Appalachian Trail with a steady supply of Green Kamut and Spirulina powders. Most days, he consumed only these green juice powders until mid-afternoon—and that was enough to get Matt over 15 miles, up and down mountains, carrying a 40-pound backpack!

If this young man could heal himself from multiple sclerosis, imagine how going green could help you move into your most healthful state.

## THE HOT THING IN GREEN FOODS

Since I have promoted the benefits of raw food, I want to make it clear that many nutrients and phytochemicals survive heat and cooking. These include powerful antioxidants like super oxide dismutase, transhydrogenase and fatty acid oxidase. Even some vegetables like spinach, and culinary herbs like onions can be better for you when cooked. In fact many foods can be consumed in their cooked or heated form and still be extremely beneficial to our bodies. Two examples are listed below.

## GREEN TEA

I get a lot of questions about green tea when I do radio call-in shows or speak at conferences. What about green tea? Does it belong in the plant-based diet? Does it have qualities that enable it to stand up and call itself truly green? Absolutely—it does. Green tea is a wonderful addition to any diet that is already green to start with and will be pretty powerful protection against every disease that plagues human beings in first world nations, especially cardiovascular disease, cancer, and Alzheimer's disease.

A large body of research shows that phytochemicals from green tea— most specifically, a catechin called *epigallocatechin gallate* (EGCG) fights cancer on all fronts. It blocks each stage of carcinogenesis—induction, where it begins; progression, where it grows; and metastasis, where it spreads throughout the body. In parts of the world where green tea consumption is highest, rates of cancer of the pancreas, small intestine, colon, stomach, breast, and lung are notably lower. Recent research has shown that green tea phytochemicals may help to prevent breast cancer recurrence. EGCG was also found to inhibit the expression of the inflammatory marker COX-2 and other indicators of inflammation in human colon cancer cells.

## GREEN TEA SEED OIL

Now another amazing use for the tea plant is emerging a true secret of the orient. Green Tea Seed Oil, which is exactly as it sounds, the oil pressed from the seeds of the tea plant. Just as the leaves contain powerful antioxidants and unique phytochemicals, so does the yield from these tiny green seeds. In fact when compared to one of my favorite tropical oils, coconut oil with a 350-375 degree smoke point, green tea seed oil can boast an amazing 475 degree smoke point. This makes it the preferred oil for the delicate Japanese culinary art of tempura style frying. Its high smoke point and delicate taste make it a cook's best friend. Perhaps the greatest benefit is reserved for its consumer because green tea seed oil is extremely healthy when compared to other cooking oils when the inflammatory impact on the body is measured. The lack of inflammatory effect is very important to note since in almost all diseases and illnesses, inflammation plays a villainous role, and cooking oils of all types create inflammatory responses in our bodies. Green tea seed oil could play an important role in food preparation in kitchens across the world for those seeking a healthier lifestyle. Many people are familiar with the Mediterranean lifestyle which includes generous amounts of fresh pressed extra virgin olive oil with a beautiful green hue. While green olive oil also has excellent anti-inflammatory qualities, they pale when compared to green tea seed oil for frying, since you should not cook on high temperatures when using olive oil. Green tea seed oil can also be added to salad dressing, mayonnaise and other oil rich foods to help improve their over-all quality and reduce their content of less healthy oils. Getting organic is very important as seeds tend to carry chemical residues.

Below are a list of benefits from the Green Tea plant:

- Inhibits angiogenesis, where cancerous tumors form new blood vessels to aid in their own growth and spread.

- Is a strong candidate for protection against skin cancer, taken orally or used topically. Green tea is one of many plant chemicals—including curcumin (from turmeric), resveratrol (from red wine and grapeseed extract), and silymarin (from milk thistle)—with promise in the skin cancer prevention department.

- Has promise as a weight-reducing aid. In cell cultures and animal models of obesity, EGCG and other green tea catechins reduce fat cell creation and the creation of the fat that goes into the fat cells. Green tea phytochemicals have been found to reduce body weight, fat absorption (in the GI tract), blood fats, cholesterol counts, blood sugars, blood insulin, and leptin levels. Green tea consumption enhances fat burning and thermogenesis (the expenditure of calories). Human studies show a reduction of body fat and body weight with regular green tea consumption.

- May help prevent Alzheimer's disease by chelating heavy metals in brain tissue (heavy metals enhance the oxidation believed to play a major role in the development of Alzheimer's). EGCG protected against the toxicity of *beta-amyloid*—the substance that accumulates in the brains of Alzheimer's disease patients—in rats.

- Has been found to effectively protect liver cells against free radicals produced during detoxification programs.

- Protects against cardiovascular disease through multiple avenues: It is protective of blood vessel walls, has antioxidant, anti-clotting, and anti-inflammatory activity, and helps to lower "bad" cholesterol counts.

- May reduce unhealthful stress responses. One Japanese animal study found that EGCG from green tea had stress-reducing effects attributable to alterations in the GABA-ergic system. When chicks were put under stressful conditions, then given EGCG injections, the chicks were calmed and their levels of stress-indicating neurotransmitters and hormones fell.

The recommended amount of green tea ranges from two to as many as ten cups a day, with most studies finding that five or more cups a day is the optimum amount for all the benefits listed above. I like to sweeten my green tea with a little agave syrup. Many flavored green teas are now available; choose one with all-natural flavorings if you don't want to drink the plain, traditional Japanese green teas.

# *Chapter Five*

## MICRO ALGAES, SPIRULINA & CHLORELLA

Viruses are not exactly alive; they're like microscopic, parasitic, multiplying aliens, like a creature in a horror movie. This helps explain why they're so hard to kill. Just when you forget about them, *they're baaack...*

In more scientific terms, a virus consists of genetic material and enzymes encased in a capsule of protein, sometimes with a lipid (fat) coating on the outside of the capsule—a missile that can pierce the armor of our cells to release its genetic "sperm." They cannot reproduce on their own, so they hijack our living cells in order to have a place to replicate and spread their progeny into more of our cells to do the same.

Viruses can't be fought with antibiotic drugs, and the antiviral drugs used to treat most common viruses are not consistently effective. After so many years of trying, modern medicine has not yet developed *truly safe* and effective drugs against the common cold, the flu virus, or the AIDS virus. Drugs commonly prescribed to treat herpes virus may help to control or shorten outbreaks, but their effects are minimal, and the potential for side effects significant.

Compared to bacteria, which are so big that they could be seen and studied by scientists in the late 1600s, viruses are miniscule and difficult to visualize.

No one was able to look at a virus under a microscope until the turn of the twentieth century. There are other more important differences; while all that's needed to test antibiotics is a culture of the bacteria—which is a relatively easy thing to do—to test antiviral drugs is more challenging. Viruses require a model using animal cells where the virus grows in the same way in which it grows in human cells. In fact, there is very little chance that drug developers will ever come up with an antiviral drug that is similar to a "broad-spectrum" antibiotic due to the unique nature of each virus; a new drug would be needed for each and every virus.

Vaccines to prevent viral diseases that once decimated significant numbers of people—mostly children and babies—have been hugely effective at prevention, but a vaccine won't help you once you've caught the virus. Besides, vaccines come with potentially adverse effects. It's just not practical or safe to give every person vaccines against every possible viral infection. The safety of giving multiple vaccines is uncertain, and we can only vaccinate against specific strains of a virus. (This is why you can still catch the flu, even if you've had the flu vaccine; it doesn't protect you from strains that are not in the vaccine.) Some of the illnesses against which most children are vaccinated are re-emerging, even in those who have had the vaccines right on schedule—most notably, whooping cough (pertussis).

Because mainstream drug-based medicine has fallen so short in finding ways to treat viral diseases, natural remedies with antiviral activity are the subject of intensive research. These remedies appear to be particularly useful in reducing the adverse effects of infection by viruses that aren't life-threatening but that put a major cramp in the lives of those who catch them. An added plus: Natural antivirals are good for many of the other things that ail modern people.

## CHLORELLA: ALL-PURPOSE HEALTH ENHANCER

In Japan, cracked-cell chlorella supplements are wildly popular, and they are making headway here in the U.S. as this plant food's health benefits become clearer.

Spirulina and chlorella are similar in that they both are chlorophyll-rich algaes. They are both rich in essential amino acids, low in fat, and high in fiber and minerals. Remember that chlorophyll is a natural anti-inflammatory, antioxidant, and wound healer that has been found to aid in normalizing the blood counts of anemic individuals, and that it has shown promise as a neutralizer of toxins.

These two types of algae contain some vitamin $B_{12}$. Some vegetarian and vegan activists claim that one can obtain all needed $B_{12}$ from a vegan diet that includes these algaes. Unfortunately, this has not proven to be the case.

Chlorella has existed on earth since the pre-Cambrian period, which means that it has been on the planet for over two billion years. It was the first form of life with a true nucleus.

The species includes any spherical, single-celled, green freshwater alga of the genus *Chlorella*. Each individual chlorella cell—a complete unicellular organism—measures 3 to 10 micrometers across. During the growth of chlorella, each of the cells can divide four times every 20 to 24 hours. Chlorella is 50 percent protein, 20 percent fat, and 20 percent carbohydrate; it also contains many minerals, vitamins, and a unique array of phytocomplexes. Science is still figuring out what exactly is in this stuff.

Along with the usual vitamin and mineral suspects found in deep green plant foods—B vitamins, carotenoids, vitamin C, magnesium—chlorella contains some potent flavonoid nutrients, including an appreciable amount of lutein, which is important for the health of the eyes. Flavonoids are plant pigments that have powerful antioxidant effects and help to strengthen the walls of blood vessels. Chlorella also contains a rare xanthophyll—a type of carotenoid that, like beta-carotene, has vitamin A activity in the body— called echinenone.

Chlorella is especially adept at making chlorophyll, and its high concentration of this substance enables it to photosynthesize—create energy from sunlight—at a very rapid clip.

## CHLORELLA: ONE ANSWER TO PESTICIDE AND HEAVY METAL TOXICITY

Each chlorella cell—its own microorganism, about the size of a human red blood cell—is encased in a tough cell wall made of hemicellulose, alpha-cellulose, protein, lipid, and an antioxidant, liver-supportive substance called *glutathione*. This cell wall has a layer of cellulose and an outer layer made up of a unique, polymerized carotenoid, and it's believed that this layer plays the greatest role in detoxification, binding to toxins and carrying them out of the body.

Compounds found in the cell walls of chlorella adhere to heavy metals in the body, including cadmium, lead, and mercury. Several research studies have shown that chlorella, when taken in proper form, reduces the body's burden of these toxic heavy metals—all of which have damaging effects on the health of the nervous and cardiovascular systems.

Unique fibers and polysaccharides in the chlorella cell wall have also been found to speed up the removal of chlorinated hydrocarbon insecticides from body tissues.

One study of rats poisoned with the insecticide chlordecone found that the half-life of the toxin (that's a measurement of the amount of time it takes for the toxin to be eliminated from the body) was reduced from 40 days to 19 days in chlorella-supplemented animals.

Another animal study, performed in Japan, examined the effects of chlorella on the effects of polychlorinated biphenyls (PCBs), a type of dioxin that is a known carcinogen. Dioxins are what's known as *persistent organic pollutants* (POPs), which means that they are stored in fats in the body and are noto-riously hard to eliminate. POPs bioaccumulate, increasing in concentration from the lowest elements of the food chain to the highest. In this experiment, rats were fed PCBs as part of one of two diets: a control diet or a 10 percent chlorella diet. The amount of dioxins excreted by the rats was measured, and—not surprisingly—the rats given chlorella excreted significantly more than the control animals.

## CHLORELLA FOR NURSING MOTHERS

One of the most frightening aspects of POPs is that their concentrations are highest in the food that's at the very pinnacle of the human food chain: human breast milk. In their book *The New Breastfeeding Diet* (McGraw-Hill, 2006), Robert Rountree, M.D., and Melissa Lynn Block recommend that nursing mothers use chlorella to gently detoxify, sending toxins out through routes other than breast milk.

How does this work? It appears that the fibrous cell wall of chlorella interferes with enterohepatic recirculation, where toxic substances are processed by the liver and sent into the GI tract for elimination—and then are reabsorbed through the walls of the large intestine to make another damaging round through the body. In some instances, the toxin has been altered into even more toxic forms through processing in the liver or by bacteria in the large intestine. Chlorella binds to these toxins in the large intestine, preventing reabsorption and moving them out of the body instead.

Liver health is essential for detoxification of toxic chemicals and drugs. An older series of studies, published in the 1970s, found that chlorella could protect the livers of rats given a potent poison called ethionine or who had sustained liver damage caused by malnutrition. The 5 percent chlorella diet also helped the rats heal more rapidly from the poisoning. The animals fed chlorella had lower levels of liver fats and cholesterol accumulation in that organ. (Fat and cholesterol accumulation in the liver indicate liver damage.)

The oxidative burst that happens when a lot of toxins come into the liver at once can cause damage to the liver, the body's most important cleansing organ, and explains the fatal nature of many types of poisonings; as the liver detox system's enzymes work to neutralize the poison in question, oxidation—a natural part of the process—escalates beyond the body's antioxidant protection mechanisms.

Chlorella's extremely high concentration of chlorophyll—higher than in any other known plant—also aids in detoxification, enhancing the operations of detox systems in the liver.

To yield the benefits of chlorella as a food, the tough cell wall must be cracked or pulverized. Consuming chlorella without a broken or crushed cell wall can cause digestive discomfort, and won't yield the same benefits to the body.

Some experts recommend that individuals with heavy metal poisoning can use 15 to 20 grams (15,000 to 20,000 milligrams) of chlorella per day. This is many times the recommended dose for general good health and prevention of disease—two to three grams per day—but no ill effects have been reported with this regimen.

## CHLORELLA GROWTH FACTOR: KEY TO STOPPING AGING?

Another special aspect of chlorella is the aptly named Chlorella Growth Factor (CGF). CGF was first isolated by a Japanese researcher from a hot water extract of chlorella, using a process called *electrophoresis*. He found that this extract promoted healthy growth in young humans and animals. The substance was later found to have immune-enhancing effects, and to promote faster tissue healing.

Found in the nucleus of each algae cell, CGF is made up of nucleic acids (DNA and RNA), amino acids (protein building blocks), carbohydrates, and vitamins. CGF also contains glutathione, an antioxidant substance that plays a crucial role in detoxification, buffering the storm of free radicals formed during the second phase of liver detoxification.

According to the research and writings of researcher Benjamin Frank, M.D., the physical deterioration that accompanies the aging process is associated with an acceleration in the breakdown of DNA and RNA within individual body cells. Dr. Frank recommends foods especially rich in nucleic acids like DNA and RNA to help rejuvenate the body's supply. High on Dr. Frank's list of DNA/RNA-rich foods: sardines. Fortunately for those who aren't fond of sardines, there is a source of DNA and RNA that is more concentrated and more palatable: chlorella, which is said to contain 17 times more RNA than those small fish.

# OTHER CHLORELLA BENEFITS

Chlorella's affinity for heavy metals has inspired some research into its potential as an environmental "cleaner-upper"—a substance that could be used to clean up heavy metals that are created as industrial wastes. In the human body, chlorella is proving useful for re-establishing balance in many of the body's systems, including the immune system, the digestive tract, the endocrine (hormonal) system, and the cardiovascular system.

## IMMUNE FUNCTION AND CANCER

Phytochemicals in chlorella stimulate interferon production in the body. Interferon is an immune factor that has cancer-fighting qualities. It increases the activity of macrophages and T-cells, both of which are important front-line defenses against cancer and infection. A glycoprotein component of chlorella showed direct anti-tumor effects in test tube studies.

## GREEN CHEMOTHERAPY?

While chlorella is more than likely to have significant protective effects against cancer—due to its detoxification and immune-boosting effects—it also is proving useful as an *adjunct* cancer therapy, used as a complement to conventional medical cancer therapies.

Studies of mice given chemotherapy drugs (including 5-fluorouracil and cyclophosphamide) have showed that adding chlorella to their regimens helps to reduce secondary infections and extend life span compared with mice given the chemo drugs without chlorella. One animal study found that mice inoculated with tumors and fed a 10 percent chlorella diet were more resistant to the subsequent growth of those tumors.

In a study at the Medical College of Virginia, patients with malignant brain tumors were given 20 grams of chlorella daily through the course of their treatment. These were patients with one of the most aggressive and deadly types of brain cancer, called malignant glioma. Although there were only minor improvements in survival time—and these were seen only in younger patients who had smaller cancers to begin with—the investigators found that the supplement improved the patients' immune function significantly. The action of immune cells that normally are suppressed by the cancer or its treatment was normalized in a significant percentage of the patients in this small study. Patients reported feeling stronger and having fewer respiratory infections and flu-like illnesses. This is especially impressive considering the fact that these patients were taking medications that greatly increase risk of opportunistic infections.

Cancer patients may take up to 20 to 30 grams of chlorella a day as a part of their treatment, but should make sure their medical team knows they're doing so. Earlier, I mentioned the Block Center for Integrative Cancer Treatment and its use of green foods as a critical aspect of cancer patients' nutritional therapy. Dr. Block told me, "For many years, I've given my patients green foods while they received chemotherapy. This led to a reduction in both their toxicity and the need to reduce the chemotherapy dosing. Reducing dosing is a big problem in cancer treatment, since it can lead to a decline in treatment benefits."

Dr. Block shared with me that he believes that patients could get through treatment more easily if they were given the right natural medicines. "Green foods are among the best kept secrets in integrative cancer treatment!" he told me.

## CHLORELLA AND CARDIOVASCULAR DISEASE

Animal studies involving rabbits and mice fed high-cholesterol diets found that chlorella supplements could delay or prevent formation of artery lesions—the blockages that lead to heart attacks and occlusive strokes.

Other research suggests that chlorella supplementation could reduce or eliminate the need for medications to control mild to moderate hypertension.

## CHLORELLA AND DIABETES

Antioxidant-rich green foods are a virtual must for people with diabetes. This condition—whether type 1, the insulin-dependent variety that usually sets in during childhood, or type 2, the non-insulin-dependent version that is linked to obesity and lack of exercise—drastically increases oxidation, inflammation, and risk of heart disease.

According to animal studies, chlorella may have specific effects helpful to those with type 2 diabetes. Taiwanese researchers found that giving chlorella to mice with type 2 diabetes—that's the version where insulin stops being able to do the work of moving sugars into cells, leading to rising blood sugars and ever-increasing insulin production as the body attempts to overcome the cells' resistance to this hormone—brought high blood sugars down. Lowering blood sugar is the first step to controlling type 2 diabetes and its devastating consequences. Further investigation revealed that this effect was due to enhanced uptake of blood sugars into the liver and muscle.

## CHLORELLA AND DIGESTIVE HEALTH

Supplementing with chlorella was strongly protective against stomach ulcers given to rats by various methods. The research team concluded that chlorella most likely worked through complex effects on the interaction of the nervous system, digestive system, and immune system, fortifying the natural protective systems of the lining of the stomach.

Ulcerative colitis affects half a million Americans. The mucous lining of the colon becomes inflamed. Bloody diarrhea, pus or mucus in the stool, and abdominal cramps are the most common symptoms. UC is a form of inflammatory bowel disease (IBD), and both causes and cures are unknown at this writing. Powerful anti-inflammatory drugs sometimes can help control UC, but they don't always work, and they carry a substantial burden of side effects.

Astoundingly, medical gastroenterology minimizes the role of diet in IBD. One textbook of gastroenterology states that "in mild to moderate ulcerative colitis, there is no need to impose general dietary restrictions." Gastroenter-ologist Ronald Hoffman, M.D., writes on this at www.consciouschoice.com:

*"This might sound, at the very least, counterintuitive to an informed layperson, who would question the dissociation between what a person eats and the condition of the selfsame ali-mentary canal through which food passes. The situation is analogous to that of a hydraulic engineer who makes no allowance for pipe corrosion susceptibility based on the acidity or chemical characteristics of the fluid the pipe conducts."*

He goes on to point out the many successes he has seen in UC patients and patients with other forms of IBD who made drastic dietary changes— usu-ally involving the elimination of grains, lactose, and sugars, and supplement-ing with good things like ginkgo biloba, licorice root, quercetin, anti-inflam-matory Chinese herbs, aloe vera, vitamins, minerals, and friendly probiotics (bacteria).

A study presented by Medical College of Virginia anatomy professor Randall E. Merchant, Ph.D., involved supplementing nine ulcerative colitis patients with 10 grams of chlorella in tablet form and 100 milliliters (mL) of liquid chlorella each day for two months. The results of the study were promising, with improvements in symptoms and clinical tests used to measure the sever-ity of the disease. Sigmoidoscopy showed decreased inflammation in the co-lon; patients reported fewer episodes of rectal bleeding; and stool frequency decreased.

With the typical Western diet, constipation and sluggish elimination are ex-tremely common. Adding chlorella as a supplement normalizes an underac-tive intestinal tract in three ways: by enhancing the natural contractions of the intestinal walls; by supplying cellulose, a form of indigestible fiber; and by promoting rapid growth of beneficial bacteria in the gut. CGF from chlo-rella helps to mend inflamed or damaged intestinal lining.

Through its enhancement of cleansing and detoxification through the bowel, chlorella has been found to improve a number of seemingly un-related conditions, including lung and bronchial issues, kidney problems, and skin conditions. When elimination is improved, fewer toxins are allowed to recirculate from the bowel back into the body. Fewer pathogenic yeasts and bacteria take root in the bowel when eliminative function is running smoothly.

## CHLORELLA AND FIBROMYALGIA

This disease involves pain in the muscles, ligaments, and tendons. The pain is chronic and comes and goes without any well-understood causes, and is usually accompanied by crushing fatigue. Fibromyalgia syndrome (FMS) has the mainstream medical community stumped.

Dr. Merchant has also researched the use of chlorella for the treatment of FMS. He and his team of researchers followed the course of 18 fibromyalgia patients over a two-month period, giving them the 10 grams plus 100 mL chlorella therapy described above. Overall, the patients reported a 22 percent reduction in the intensity of their pain.

A 35-year-old mother of three tried chlorella after her diagnosis of chronic fatigue syndrome and fibromyalgia. She took 20 tablets of chlorella a day and within a few months, she felt significantly better, with more energy, less pain, and greater resistance to infection.

## CHLORELLA AND COLDS AND FLU

About half of the crew of a cruise ship—almost 1,000 sailors—were given two grams of chlorella per day for the duration of a training cruise from Japan to Australia and back. The other half did not take chlorella during that 95-day voyage. Sailors who used chlorella had about 30 percent fewer cases of cold and flu compared to control subjects. *Chlon A*, a substance which has been isolated from the nucleic material of chlorella, was probably to thank for the infection-fighting benefit; it stimulates the production of interferon, an immune factor that promotes an overall boost in immune activity.

## CHLORELLA AND AUTISM

Autism rates have risen dramatically in recent years. Diagnosis of this developmental disorder is particularly high in children born between the years of 1987 and 1992, according to an ABC news report on a study published in the academic journal *Pediatrics*. This disorder is characterized by inability to socialize and communicate, along with repetitive, obsessive, or self-abusive behaviors. Usually, it strikes by the age of three and in most cases hangs on for life. Other milder autism-related disorders, such as Asperger's syndrome—which fell into the public eye upon publication of the best-selling novel, *The Curious Incident of the Dog in the Night-Time*, in 2004—are also on the rise.

At a meeting called on this subject in 2000, physician Stephanie Cave of Baton Rouge, Louisiana, spoke about her experiences treating autistic children—over 400 of them. No therapy worked as well for as many children, she told the group, as mercury detoxification. Parents of autistic kids at that meeting, and other physicians, seconded Dr. Cave's remarks.

Other theories about autism have to do with poor intestinal absorption of nutrients or food sensitivities; it's widely agreed that these issues must be dealt with through dietary changes—changes that just happen to be similar to those I recommend in my Plant Based Nutrition Programs. Another theory speculates that antioxidant deficiencies play a role in the disorder. Lab tests have found deficiencies of important antioxidants in autistic children at the cellular level. Some agents used to help detoxify mercury also happen to be powerful antioxidants—including a chelating agent (a synthetic amino acid that "grabs" metals and helps move them out of the body) called DMSA. Chlorella is also a chelator, and it also happens to contain dozens of antioxidant plant chemicals.

Autistic children often will only eat a very limited number of foods, and their overall nutritional intake can suffer and potentially their problems can worsen as a result. It's hard enough to get a child without autism to eat healthfully in today's refined-carbohydrate-and-junk-food-saturated environment—with an autistic child, it can be an unwinnable battle. Supplementing the child's diet with a safe, mercury-detoxifying, antioxidant-rich food like chlorella can make a big difference in that child's nutritional intake. In some cases, it can bring about significant improvements in their symptoms.

Bianca's three-year-old son had been diagnosed with regressive autism, and with a restricted diet (no gluten—the protein in many grains; and no casein—milk protein), cod-liver oil, probiotics, and some other supplements, her son got worse, then better, slowly. But until she added chlorella to his supplement plan, she didn't see dramatic improvement. In only a few months, her son went from speaking only 3 words to speaking more than 70 words, and began to speak in sentences for the first time. Social skills, imaginary play, and potty training all began to majorly improve. She reports that he no longer seems to be autistic.

Another parent reported that her son's autistic symptoms were reversed with a combination of low-grain, organic, fresh-food diet and daily chlorella. The child became more adept at interacting with peers; his physical skills improved; and school staff members were completely blown away by his progress, predicting that the child would soon no longer need special education services. Some of these professionals had been working with autistic children for decades.

Considering the combination of factors that appear to contribute to autism, the helpful effects of chlorella for autistic children are unsurprising. It aids in mercury detoxification; it contains high concentrations of antioxidants; and is packed with vitamins and minerals in highly bioavailable forms, which makes it ideal for filling in nutritional gaps in the diets of autistic children.

For more detailed information on mercury detoxification and nutrition protocols for autistic children, go to the Web site of the Autism Research Institute, home of Defeat Autism Now! (DAN!), at http://www.autismwebsite.com/ARI/dan/dan.htm.

## HANGOVERS

Japanese researchers gave study subjects four to five grams of chlorella before having them drink varying amounts of alcohol. The chlorella reduced hangover incidence by 96 percent—most likely through enhancement of the liver's ability to detoxify the alcohol.

## HOW CHLORELLA IS CULTIVATED AND PROCESSED

This plant, whose name is derived from the Greek *chloros* (green) and *ella* (small), is usually cultivated in large, freshwater pools containing mineral-rich water, in places where sunlight exposure is optimal. A strict schedule of inspections and steps for maintaining a monoculture—an algal growth that contains no potentially toxic strains of algae—is followed. No pesticides or chemical additives are used.

After harvesting, the chlorella requires processing to break down its cell wall. A patented process has been developed to break down the cell walls without heat, or chemicals—protecting its enzyme content and nutritional value.

# SPIRULINA: NATURE'S MOST BALANCED SOURCE OF NUTRITION

Spirulina is one form of blue-green algae, the planet's most ancient form of plant life. Blue-green algae is still an important foundation of the food chain, feeding the smallest insects and sea creatures that are themselves food for slightly larger animals. It is extremely nutrient-dense, containing high concentrations of chlorophyll (the pigment that makes green plants green, and that transmutes the sun's energy into food within the plant), vitamins, minerals, and amino acids. Spirulina has a soft, malleable cell wall that is easily broken down in the digestive system. Spirulina's name comes from the spiral shape of each individual spirulina cell.

So nutrient-dense is this algae, so quick to grow, and so hardy—many blue-green algaes can grow anywhere, in brackish or alkaline water, in polar ice caps, and in scorching hot springs—some experts believe that it could be used as a whole-food multi-nutrient supplement for populations at risk for malnutrition or starvation. Spirulina doubles its biomass in two to five days, and can be cultivated on land where nothing else will grow. In the same amount of space, spirulina yields over 20 times more protein than soybeans and 400 times more protein than beef.

## POND SCUM...NOT!

It's sometimes said that spirulina is nothing but "pond scum." The truth is that there are algaes that grow in fresh water that are *not* spirulina and are toxic. There are wild monocultures of spirulina in certain parts of the world that can be eaten safely, but only an expert eye can tell which cultures are edible. It is important to use only spirulina that is carefully cultivated in pure water under ideal conditions, and we ensure that no toxic algal blooms enter the picture. Go to www.pureplanet.com for more info.

Spirulina that goes into the making of nutritional supplements is usually grown in outdoor tanks. The most commonly used varieties are *Spirulina maxima* (grown in Mexico) and *Spirulina platensis* (grown in Hawaii).

In some lakes in Africa, Mexico, and Central and South America, spirulina grows wild and has long been a food source, made into sun-dried cakes or bouillon. It was used as a food by Aztecs hundreds of years ago. It's been postulated that the "manna from heaven" mentioned in the Bible was flat cakes of dried spirulina.

Spirulina contains 10 times more beta-carotene than carrots. It also contains high concentrations of gamma-linoleic acid (GLA), an anti-inflammatory omega-6 fatty acid. GLA is useful for relief of premenstrual symptoms, and promotes improved skin health. It's also important for prenatal nutrition, and passes into breast milk to provide good nutrition for the nursing baby. The anti-inflammatory effects of GLA and *phycocyanin*, the blue-green pigment unique to blue-green algaes like spirulina, could explain why many people attest to spirulina's ability to relieve joint pains and body aches.

Users often report dramatic improvements in their energy levels. Athletes use it to improve performance and endurance for training, and generally find that it also aids in faster recovery from tough workouts. Spirulina is rich in iron and magnesium, and is an excellent source of trace minerals. It is nature's multivitamin!

Like chlorella, spirulina is wildly popular in Japan, used by many as a food supplement. It is cheaper to grow and process than chlorella, and so has more promise for reducing worldwide malnutrition. In fact, the United Nations and World Health Organization have both recommended spirulina as a safe food supplement for children. One study of West African children found enhanced weight gain when a teaspoon of spirulina powder was added to their daily diets.

A few animal studies suggest that spirulina promotes the formation and maturation of red blood cells, which carry oxygen throughout the body. High levels of chlorophyll and iron are the likely reasons for these results.

Spirulina is particularly well suited for people who have poor digestion. It has a soft cell wall made up of proteins, polysaccharides, and enzymes that is very easy for even a compromised digestive system to break down. It's an ideal supplement for the very elderly, the very sick, and the very young.

## PHYCOCYANINS: BLUE-GREEN PIGMENTS

Spirulina contains a unique blue-green pigment called phycocyanin, which gives the plants a bluish tinge. Phycocyanin and related compounds have been found to help maintain balanced immune system function. In lab studies, phycocyanin inhibited the formation of inflammatory chemicals by the immune system. Like the drugs Vioxx and Celebrex, this plant chemical inhibits the COX-2 enzyme—a major player in excess inflammation. Other research has found that phycocyanins block angiogenesis, the formation of new blood vessels to feed cancerous tumors.

Spirulina has been researched extensively for its potential to improve immune function. Those blue and green pigments can rev up the action of white blood cells in engulfing and digesting pathogens, and it has been found to increase the action of natural killer cells (anti-cancer, antiviral). Spirulina enhances antibody function (antibodies are the immune factors that are produced in response to infection or vaccination) and may help the body to resist food allergies.

Like red marine algae, spirulina helps reduce the virulence of viruses in the body. In test tube studies, the algae reduced replication of cytomegalovirus, measles virus, mumps virus, a strain of flu, and the virus that causes herpes simplex 1. Spirulina supplementation prolongs the lives of animals infected with HSV-1 (the herpes simplex 1 virus).

## IMMUNITY AND BLUE-GREEN ALGAE

Researchers the world over are studying the potential of algaes for treatment of the HIV virus. Several compounds with HIV-inhibiting actions have been isolated from algae, including one called *cyanovirin-N*, and glycolipids and complex carbohydrates (polysaccharides) unique to blue-green algae. In one study, enhancements in immune function lasted for up to five weeks after the last dose of spirulina!

## SPIRULINA VS. CANCER

Indian researchers found that animals with cancer could fight it better with the aid of spirulina. At a dosage level of 500 milligrams per kilogram of body weight, tumor burden was halved compared to that of control animals who received no spirulina. An animal study of skin cancer found that lower doses (250 mg/kg) reduced tumor burden to one-fourth that of controls.

Leukoplakia, a precancerous mouth condition, responds well to spirulina treatment. A study performed in India found that these whitish patches, often found in the mouths of tobacco chewers and smokers, could be minimized or completely regressed with the use of one gram of spirulina per day. A year later, long after the supplements had been discontinued, 55 percent of the men were still free of leukoplakia.

Studies find that spirulina helps maintain better immune system function in mice and dogs undergoing chemotherapy and radiation treatments. Since the adverse immune system effects of these therapies are a major issue in cancer patients—even leading to the patient's death from infection— spirulina could help when people require these aggressive treatments.

Interestingly, spirulina was used in Russia to treat victims—especially children—of the nuclear accident at Chernobyl. The victims' bone marrow, compromised in blood cell production by radiation, seemed to better bounce back to its proper function when spirulina was administered.

# *Chapter Six*

## CRUCIFEROUS VEGETABLES, LEAFY GREENS, & SPROUTS

"Eat your greens," your mother said. If you were like most kids, you did your best to push them around on your plate, bury them under your potatoes, feed them to the dog—*anything* to avoid actually eating them. The face of a child who doesn't like greens who finally caves to parental pressure to eat them is such a perfect picture of taste-bud rebellion, it can be hard not to laugh in the face of her suffering.

As adults, most of our taste buds have changed enough that we actually enjoy the tastes and textures of at least some green foods. The more of them we include in our diets, the better, because each green food has its own unique set of gifts. There's a lot more to green food than lettuce and the occasional serving of overcooked broccoli. Hopefully, as you read on, you'll be motivated to try a few you've never tried, even if they make you wrinkle your nose a bit at first!

When Hippocrates said, "Thy food shall be thy remedy," he was obviously thinking of the vegetable kingdom. Green vegetables are packed with antioxidants and anti-inflammatory chemicals, as well as a few newly discovered plant chemicals that have specific and potent protective actions against cancer and heart disease. Green vegetables are also loaded with fiber, chlorophyll, vitamins, and trace minerals. Sprouts are especially wonderful because they're still *alive* when you eat them—they're full of energy that translates to energy you can feel in your body. When the body becomes too acidic—a result of overeating sweets, starches, proteins and processed foods in general—it's the alkalinity of vegetables that best helps us neutralize the acid and bring our bodies back into a state of balance.

In this chapter, you'll learn all there is to learn about the most highly nutritious vegetables cultivated by human beings: the cruciferous vegetables, including broccoli, cauliflower, and cabbage; the leafy greens; and the tiny package of powerful life energy that is a sprouted bean, nut, or seed.

## THE CRUCIFEROUS VEGETABLES

*Cruciferous* vegetables are those that belong to the mustard family: cabbages, brussels sprouts, cresses, radishes, turnips, and the best-known of this family, broccoli and cauliflower. They are also known as *Brassica* vegetables. These terms are interchangeable, and yes, this family of vegetables includes the plant from which mustard is made.

Mustard has been used since Biblical times as both a medicine and a condiment, and is a part of a huge family of plants. Most of the crucifers have a biting, peppery, or pungent taste. The petals of the flowers on this family of plants form a Maltese cross—a cross with arms of equal length—said to symbolize the sun. This is why they were originally called *cruciferae*, for "cross-bearer." Botanists have classified over 3,000 species of plants as crucifers.

The mustard family vegetables, including watercress, radishes, turnips and cabbages, have been grown since ancient times. A wild cabbage with many fleshy leaves and no head—a distant cousin of kale—is still found along the coastal cliffs of Europe. From this wild ancestor, cabbage, cauliflower, brussels sprouts, broccoli, kohlrabi, kale and collard, rape, turnip and rutabagas were all cultivated over the centuries.

A cabbage head is really just an enlarged outer bud that does not open. In kale and collards, this bud opens. The small heads of brussels sprouts are side buds. Cauliflower and broccoli are modified flowers. We eat the swollen stem of kohlrabi, the root of turnip and rutabaga, and their green, leafy tops. These *Brassica* vegetables grow in the winter, the darker months of the year.

Most members of the *Brassicaceae* family share a suite of phytonutrients referred to as *glucosinolates*. Studies show that the glucosinolates help to eliminate carcinogenic toxins in the body and encourage self-destruction of pre-cancerous cells. More on this a bit later in the chapter.

## KING CABBAGE

Now, let's take a closer look at the head of this family—one of the most versatile and richest vegetables of all time: cabbage. Cabbages come in many colors, shapes, and sizes. Since they've been around for so long, they are the subject of lots of colorful folklore.

Cabbage was one of the most coveted plants in medieval gardens; it's been around since antiquity. The Germans and Celts were fervent cultivators of all species of cabbage. The Romans believed that cabbage could cure melancholia, and they used it to counteract the effects of too much alcohol.

Early immigrants to North America wanted to bring along something of their homeland. Since space was a problem, they often tucked a garden cutting or a handful of native seeds or roots into their bags or pocket. This is probably how early immigrants brought the common cabbage to America. It's believed that we have Russian and Irish immigrants to thank for introducing this vegetable to the Atlantic shores of the new world. Chinese immigrants brought the Oriental versions of cabbage—including napa and bok choy—to Pacific shores.

Enter the railroad. As Irish and Russian settlers moved westward, they took their cabbage plants with them. With the expansion eastward of the American railroad system, Chinese workers edged their favorite vegetable along with iron

THE GREEN FOODS BIBLE

and steel, coal, wood and smoke. Soon, the two, East and West, met, and cabbage became one of the most cultivated vegetables in the New World.

Generally speaking, there are three main types of cabbage: white, red, and Savoy.

- White cabbage—which is really pale green—is the most common. Eaten either raw or cooked, white cabbage is the most important of all head cabbage species; it's the one from which cole slaw and sauerkraut are made.

- Savoy is "curly" cabbage, with leaves that are ruffled, deeply ridged, and deeply veined. Its taste is a bit milder and its texture softer. It can be used for salads or stuffed. This one is richest of all its cabbage cousins in the carotenoid nutrient beta-carotene.

- Red cabbage has more than twice as much vitamin C as green. (On the other hand, green cabbage has about twice as much folate as the red.) It has a smaller, very firm head and a slightly sweet taste.

Cabbages contain more vitamin C than oranges. They're a superlative source of essential minerals, including potassium and calcium, and contain abundant vitamin $B_1$ and $B_2$. The outer leaves contain more vitamin E and calcium than the inner leaves. Making cabbage into sauerkraut—a technique extolled by raw foodists as excellent for improving this vegetable's digestibility and the bioavailability of its nutrients—promotes healthy intestinal flora and strengthens the intestines.

Now that you're convinced that eating cabbage is a good idea, here are two things to keep in mind. First, cabbages should not be sliced until they are ready to be used. Tearing the cell walls by cutting releases enzymes that hasten oxidation and the destruction of vitamin C, effectively lowering its antioxidant content. Second, eating raw cabbage every day can suppress the activity of the thyroid gland; in other words, cabbage (and other crucifers, including broccoli and cauliflower) in their raw state are *goitrogenic*.

French phytotherapist Jean Valnet has devoted an entire chapter in his book, *Heal Yourself with Vegetables, Fruit and Cereals*, to cabbage and its healing and life-enhancing properties. He shines light on cabbage's ability to heal ulcers—which he attributes, in part, to cabbage's content of gelatinous soluble fiber. Soluble fiber, also known as *mucilage*, has a coating, soothing effect on damaged areas of the gastrointestinal tract. The anti-ulcer effects of cabbage have also been attributed to a phytochemical Valnet calls "vitamin U," which protects mucous membranes. Cabbages are a good source of vitamin K, which aids in proper blood clotting—a vitamin important for the prevention of GI bleeds that can occur with ulcers. (For ulcer therapy, Valnet recommends enzyme-rich raw cabbage juice or freshly chopped raw cabbage.)

In his book, Dr. Valnet relates a story from the 1880s: A young man fell from his coach and his leg was run over by the wheel. The two village doctors who examined him following the accident told him his leg would have to be amputated, but the village priest told the young man's mother to cover his leg with cabbage leaves. She followed his advice late in the afternoon, and by nightfall, the boy's pain was alleviated enough that he could sleep. The next day, the doctors arrived to perform the amputation, but found that the boy's leg was much improved. Within eight days, the young man was able to resume his regular work.

## MORE ON VITAMIN U

"Vitamin U"—not really a vitamin—is thought to aid in the healing of skin ulcers and ulcers in the digestive tract. It's also known as *cabagin*; in scientific terms, it's referred to as methylmethionine sulfonium chloride. This chemical is to thank (or, perhaps, to blame) for the strong odor of cabbage. Its title of "vitamin U" is derived from the success that has been achieved with its use as an ulcer therapy.

The traditional use of raw cabbage juice as the treatment of choice for stomach ulcers has been extensively confirmed by scientific research, particularly in Russia and other countries of the former Soviet Union.

The aroma of cabbage comes, in large part, from its sulfur content. If you have visited a hot sulfur spring in your lifetime, you know that the experience of those rejuvenating and healing waters can be somewhat spoiled by the powerful rotten-egg smell.

Our bodies need sulfur—it builds bones and connective tissues, and is vital for healthy skin. Some sulfur preparations, such as *methylsulfonymethane* (MSM), are widely used as nutritional supplements to support skin, bone, and hair health. Some respected medical experts even recommend its use as a natural medicine for pain.

Sulfur has disinfectant and tonifying properties; this could explain why traditional medicine often prescribed cabbage or other sulfur-rich foods (including garlic) to help heal or ward off respiratory ailments. Cabbage also soothes and helps to heal eczema.

## CABBAGE ISN'T JUST FOR EATING—IT'S FOR WEARING, TOO

Amanda loved their house in the country. She regularly retreated to it to get away from the chaos and stress of city life and her demanding and stressful job as a journalist. Many times she spent whole weekends in bed, suffering from horrible migraines. Then one day her neighbor told her about the virtues of Savoy cabbage leaves for relieving headaches.

Although she has since quit her stressful job in the city, her vegetable patch offers a variety of natural remedies, and cabbage holds a special place of honor. Now as soon as she feels a headache coming on, she brings in a head of Savoy cabbage from her garden. She lays a few leaves out on her table and rolls them with a rolling pin to flatten them and break up big veins. Then she applies them to her head like a helmet, puts a band around them to hold them in place, and lies down. Within anywhere from 15 minutes to two hours, she's back on her feet and that headache nothing but a memory.

Another topical use for cabbage leaves: Nursing mothers experiencing engorgement or mastitis (infection of the milk ducts) are often advised by midwives or doulas to use cabbage leaves as a remedy. White cabbage leaves, flattened with a rolling pin, are placed inside the bra and changed every two hours.

Not sure how to add cabbage to your daily fare? A couple of suggestions:

- Mix brown rice with raw cashews, shredded red cabbage, and chunks of tofu. Add two or three tablespoons of oil and vinegar dressing and toss thoroughly to make a delicious rice salad. Add grated raw beets, carrots, crunchy sprouts (like those from chickpeas, green peas, or pumpkin seeds) or other vegetables you enjoy.

- Pile shredded white or Savoy cabbage instead of lettuce into tacos

- Add shredded cabbage to soups for great flavor and added nutrition.

## CRUCIFEROUS CANCER PROTECTION

New research has greatly advanced scientists' understanding of just how *Brassica* family vegetables help prevent cancer. When these vegetables are cut, chewed or digested, a sulfur-containing compound called *sinigrin* is brought into contact with the enzyme *myrosinase*. This releases glucose and breakdown products, including highly reactive compounds called *isothiocyanates*.

Isothiocyanates are central to inducing the liver's Phase II enzymes, which detoxify carcinogens. Recent research conducted at the Institute for Food Research in the UK shows one of these compounds, *allyl isothiocyanate*, also inhibits mitosis (cell division) and stimulates apoptosis (programmed cell death) in human tumor cells. The IFR team, led by Ian Johnson, demonstrated that isothiocyanate disrupts the cell division of colon cancer cells. Their research was published in the July 2004 issue of the journal *Carcinogenesis*.

## BROCCOLI

Broccoli may just be the first of the family to be developed from the wild species of kale or cabbage and cultivated by the Romans. It was introduced in England in the early sixteenth century and referred to as "Italian asparagus" or "sprout cauliflower." Broccoli came to the United States only recently. It was grown in the 1800s, but didn't become popular until the 1930s. Italian-Americans were the first to popularize what they originally called "little sprouts" in Italian. Like other cruciferous vegetables, broccoli contains phy-tochemicals—the antioxidant *sulforaphane* and natural compounds known as the *indoles* (best-known is *indole-3-carbinol*)—which have significant anti-cancer effects.

Research on indole-3-carbinol shows that it helps deactivate a break-down product of the female hormone estrogen (*4-hydroxyestrone*) that promotes tumor growth, especially in estrogen-sensitive breast cells. At the same time, it increases the level of *2-hydroxyestrone*, a form of estrogen said to offer protection against cancer.

Indole-3-carbinol has been shown to suppress not only breast tumor cell growth, but also cancer cell metastasis (the movement of cancerous cells to other parts of the body). Scientists have found that sulforaphane boosts the activity of the body's detoxification enzymes by altering gene expression (the process that translates the information coded into the genes into cell structures and processes). It helps your body dispose of potentially carcinogenic substances more quickly. When researchers at Johns Hopkins studied the effect of sulforaphane on tumor formation in lab animals, animals given sulforaphane had fewer tumors, and the tumors they did develop grew more slowly and were smaller in size.

Like other members of the cabbage family, broccoli is an excellent source of vitamin C (excellent for the immune system), carotene (produces vitamin A), folic acid (helps protect against birth defects, reinforces cell growth), and dietary fiber (promotes healthy bowel function). It is also a good source of other vitamins, minerals and trace elements.

Broccoli isn't everyone's favorite food, but it's an important green food to include in your diet. Try it a few different ways: lightly steamed with garlic butter and a sprinkling of flavorful cheese; raw, with yogurt dip; stir-fried with ginger, garlic, and sesame oil; or in a casserole.

One friend of mine makes a spectacular broccoli salad with a head of fresh, organic broccoli, one half of a chopped red onion, and a dressing made with two tablespoons of apple cider vinegar, and agave nectar or brown rice syrup to taste, and 3/4 cup of homemade mayonnaise (the old-fashioned kind, which she makes fresh with organic eggs and extra-virgin olive oil). Even the most die-hard broccoli disdainer has been seen gobbling this salad down.

## CAULIFLOWER

Mark Twain called cauliflower "cabbage with a college education." Cauliflower's elegant appearance has earned it the title of most refined cruciferous vegetable. It stays white because its leaves shield the growing florets from the sun. This winter crop tastes best during the height of its harvest season, which runs from December to March.

Like broccoli, cauliflower contains powerful cancer-fighting compounds. These compounds, glucosinolates (sulforaphane) and thiocyanates (isothiocyanate), increase the liver's ability to neutralize potentially toxic substances.

When the liver cannot quickly and properly dispose of toxic substances in the body, these substances can damage cell membranes and even the DNA within the cell nucleus. This can cause a chain reaction that could lead to carcinogenesis—cell deregulation and uncontrolled growth. Several enzymes found in cauliflower help the body's detoxifying process, including *glutathione transferase*, *glucuronosyl transferase*, and *quinone reductase*.

If anyone you love is dealing with prostate cancer, you may want to serve them cauliflower with turmeric, the bright-yellow relative of the ginger root that gives curry powder its vivid color. Researchers have attributed the low incidence of prostate cancer among men in India to diets rich in curried *Brassicaceae* family vegetables.

Scientists tested the effects of turmeric—which is a concentrated source of the phytonutrient curcumin—plus a phytochemical abundant in cruciferous vegetables, known as *phenethyl isothiocyanates*, on the growth of human prostate cancer cells that had been implanted in lab mice. When tested singly, both phenethyl isothiocyanate and curcumin greatly slowed the growth of the human prostate cancer cells. In mice with established prostate cancer tumors, neither phenethyl isothiocyanate nor curcumin alone had a protective effect, but when combined, they caused a significant reduction in both tumor growth and prostate cancer metastasis in the test animals.

Researchers concluded that the combination of cruciferous vegetables plus curcumin could be effective in not only preventing prostate cancer, but in inhibiting metastasis of established prostate cancers. Best of all, the combination of cauliflower spiced with turmeric is quite tasty!

A few suggestions for preparing cauliflower:

- Cut cauliflower florets in quarters and allow them to sit for 5 to 10 minutes so that the phenethyl isothiocyanates have time to develop. These compounds form when crucifer vegetables are cut, but stop forming when they are heated. Sprinkle with turmeric or curry powder and sauté at medium heat in a few tablespoons of vegetable broth for five minutes. Remove from the heat and top with olive oil, sea salt and pepper to taste.

- For a heartier cauliflower dish, heat 1/4 cup butter, ghee (clarified butter, used in Indian cooking), or coconut oil, in a deep skillet at medium heat. Add a finely chopped onion, two tablespoons of curry powder, and a julienned one-inch piece of ginger and cook until the onion is soft. Stir in two tablespoons of tomato paste and a cup of water, then the cauliflower, cut into florets, and three cups of canned garbanzo beans (chickpeas). Reduce the heat to medium-low, cover, and simmer for 15 to 20 minutes, until it's soft and the sauce is thickened, then enjoy.

- Try adding a handful of celery leaves or 1/2 teaspoon celery seeds to cauliflower cooking water. This helps reduce the typical cabbage odor.

- Add a little lemon juice to cauliflower cooking water to prevent reactions between the vegetable's phytochemicals and the iron in the cookware— reactions that can turn the cauliflower an unappetizing brown.

# BRUSSELS SPROUTS

Brussels sprouts: You either love 'em or hate 'em. Originally, they were cultivated in large quantities in Belgium—that's where their name comes from—in the late 1500s. They are thought to have been cultivated in Italy in Roman times. Americans didn't partake of this fascinating vegetable until the 1800s.

Like other members of the cabbage family, brussels sprouts are a cool weather crop. Unlike cabbage, which stores well, brussels sprouts, cauliflower and (especially) broccoli should not be stored for more than a few days. These three crucifers need to be kept in the vegetable bin of the refrigerator, wrapped in a sealable plastic bag. Add a couple of drops of water to the bag to delay yellowing and spoilage. Once these vegetables have begun to yellow, their life-enhancing properties are pretty much lost.

Brussels sprouts are high in protein. But the protein is incomplete— lacking the full spectrum of essential amino acids. A serving of whole grains can easily provide the amino acids that are missing from these little cabbages.

Detractors of brussels sprouts are usually put off by their bitterness. It's interesting to note that cutting crosses in their stems before cooking will remove some of that bitter flavor. Once you've done this, soak them in ice water, then throw them into boiling water for 7 to 10 minutes. Halt the cooking process by returning them to the ice water. Properly prepared, fresh brussels sprouts have a delicate taste that even kids can learn to like.

Brussels sprouts are also great oven-roasted. Toss a pound of sprouts in three tablespoons of extra-virgin olive oil, a teaspoon of sea salt, and a teaspoon of freshly ground pepper and roast on an oiled sheet pan for 30 to 35 minutes, turning once or twice. They'll get brown on the outside and tender inside. Grate some good Romano cheese over them just before serving.

# IN CASE YOU ARE NOT CONVINCED...

Although George H. W. Bush refused to eat his broccoli, the evidence in favor of the nutritional benefits of this and other *Brassica* vegetables might have helped him forego the pork rinds and munch on broccoli florets instead!

- Cruciferous vegetables are excellent sources of vitamin C, the body's primary water-soluble antioxidant. Vitamin C supports immune function and the manufacture of collagen, a protein that forms the ground substance of body structures including the skin, connective tissue, cartilage, and tendons. An important study conducted on close to 20,000 men and women in England found that people with the highest levels of vitamin C had half the risk of dying from heart disease, stroke or cancer. Risk of dying from heart disease was reduced by 71 percent in men and 59 percent for women in the group with the highest vitamin C levels.

- And vitamin C may also help you maintain healthy joints—but it looks like you may need to get it from food instead of lab-created single-nutrient supplements. One study published in July of 2004 suggests that high doses of supplemental vitamin C can make osteoarthritis worse in guinea pigs; another study indicates that vitamin C-rich foods, such as crucifer family vegetables, protect against inflammatory polyarthritis, a form of rheumatoid arthritis involving two or more joints. These findings, presented in the Annals of the Rheumatic Diseases, covered more than 20,000 subjects who kept diet journals. Subjects who consumed the lowest amounts of vitamin C-rich foods were more than three times more likely to develop arthritis than those who consumed the higher amounts.

- Cruciferous vegetables contain elevated amounts of beta-carotene—a vitamin A precursor—both of which play important roles in fending off infection and promoting resilient, glowing skin.

- *Brassica* vegetables are all also rich in folate, a B vitamin that is essential in DNA synthesis. Without folic acid, the nervous system cells of a developing fetus do not divide properly. Deficiency of folic acid during pregnancy has been linked to several birth defects, including neural tube defects like spina bifida. Despite folic acid's wide occurrence in food (its name comes from the Latin word *folium*, meaning "foliage," because it's found in green leafy vegetables), folic acid deficiency is the most common vitamin deficiency in the world.

- Adding these vegetables to your diet also increases your fiber intake. All the crucifers add both soluble and insoluble fiber to your diet—both of which fill you up and satisfy hunger more quickly. Fiber also prevents intestinal diseases like diverticulosis and colon cancer, in two ways: by nourishing the cells that line the walls of the colon, and by helping to create large, soft, bulky stools that are easy to eliminate.

## THE VITAMIN A DEBATE

Vitamin A, also known as retinol, is found in its preformed state in animal foods, including fish and organ meats. But even strict vegetarians can get adequate vitamin A; plants contain beta-carotene and other carotenoid nutrients that the body can convert into vitamin A, provided certain conditions are fulfilled.

Beta-carotene is *not* vitamin A. You might read in health books or articles that vegetables like carrots and spinach contain vitamin A, or that beta-carotene is like vitamin A. The truth: Vitamin A and the carotenes are very different, despite the fact that some carotenes can be converted into vitamin A. Both types of nutrients have value and play important—but different—roles in the body.

Vitamin A is a fat-soluble vitamin—the first vitamin discovered. In the 1930s, researchers described vitamin A as the "anti-infective vitamin," since it's intimately involved in the health of the mucous membranes and in fighting off infections. It's also vital for good eye health and night vision. The carotenes are a large family of plant pigments that are water- soluble and have powerful antioxidant, cardiovascular-protective, and cancer-preventive effects. Carotenes are a major reason why a diet rich in vegetables is so health-promoting.

The conversion from carotene to vitamin A takes place in the intestines, as long as bile salts—made in the liver and stored in the gallbladder, from which they are pumped when fat passes through the GI tract—are present. It follows that fat must be eaten with the carotenes to stimulate bile secretion in order to take advantage of their vitamin A activity. But many people—including infants and people with hypothyroidism (underactive thyroid), gall bladder problems, or diabetes—are either incapable of converting carotene to vitamin A or have difficulty converting it.

Lastly, the body does not convert carotene to vitamin A very efficiently. It takes roughly six units of carotene to make one unit of vitamin A. In other words, if you eat a sweet potato (containing about 25,000 units of beta-carotene), the body will only convert about 4,000 units of vitamin A when conditions are optimal.

If you aren't getting plenty of carotenes in your daily diet—along with a fat source like butter, avocado, nuts, or seeds—you may not want to rely on plant sources for vitamin A. Eating lots of colorful vegetables and fruits at each meal (or using a whole plant food supplement like those made by Pure Planet) will supply your body with plenty of carotenes, but animal foods and fats (if you are not vegan) ensure that you are getting enough preformed vitamin A. Butter and full-fat dairy foods, especially from pastured cows, are good vitamin A sources. Fatty fish and cod liver oil are also good sources of preformed vitamin A.

## LEAFY GREENS

Some overlap exists between the categories of cruciferous vegetables and leafy greens. Kale, collard greens, and bok choy, for example, are often referred to as leafy greens, but they are also crucifers. Rather than get into a detailed discussion of the botanical nomenclature, I'll let that issue go with a mention. It isn't necessary to split hairs about which greens go in which classification, because you should eat them *all!*

The leafy greens are right up there near the top of the list of the world's most nourishing, protective foods. And they might help us think more clearly and stay sharp in school.

Research conducted at Tufts University's Friedman School of Nutrition Science and Policy suggests that folate—which is especially abundant in leafy green vegetables—may protect against cognitive decline in older adults. Ongoing studies, including a few from the Linus Pauling Institute at Oregon State University, conclude that folate plays an essential role for normal brain function.

## KALE

This leafy green comes in a rainbow of colors and can be downright delicious. Unfortunately, in a culture where highly processed, melt-in-your-mouth treats are never more than a short drive away, its faintly bitter taste and unique texture is—to put it mildly—underappreciated.

Kale is by far one of the healthiest greens for your bones. One cup of cooked kale contains whopping amounts of vitamin K, a nutrient that helps support healthy bone formation. This leafy green vegetable also contains manganese, which promotes bone density, and it is also high in calcium. Kale is the top leafy green source of the carotenoids *lutein* and *zeaxanthin*, which promote eye health. These carotenoids are the same ones found in the retinas of the eyes, where they shield those delicate surfaces from the damaging ultraviolet rays of the sun. It follows that eating lots of kale may help lower the risk of age-related macular degeneration (a blinding eye disease) and cataracts.

Kale, like other members of its family, is a rich source of cancer-preventive nutrients, including vitamin C, sulforaphane, and indoles. Together, the vitamin $B_2$ and $B_6$ in kale work as catalysts to assist healthy heart functioning. And let's not forget the fiber content in kale, which has been shown to help reduce cholesterol levels. Fiber-rich kale is also useful in keeping blood sugar levels under control. Finally, kale's fiber binds to cancer-causing chemicals, keeping them away from the cells lining the colon. This fiber provides yet another line of protection from colon cancer, reducing risk of constipation, diarrhea and irritable bowel syndrome in the process.

Raw kale is better than you think. Try preparing it this way: Remove the stems of a bunch of fresh dinosaur or red Russian kale. Rip the leaves into bite-sized pieces. Slice a quarter of a red onion, very thinly; also slice or julienne a zucchini. Mix all of these ingredients together, then add dressing: 3/4 cup olive oil, 1/2 cup lemon juice, and a teaspoon of salt. Pour the dressing over the leaves and massage it in—the lemon juice and oil will break down the kale. Add a clove of crushed garlic and two avocadoes (ripe but firm), cut into chunks.

If you prefer your kale cooked, you can try adding it to soups—it's especially good in bean soups. Or, you can sauté some garlic in olive oil, then add a pound of kale (remove stems first) with a couple of tablespoons of water. Cover and allow the kale to wilt. Add a dash of tamari and sesame seeds if you like Asian flavors.

Use kale in quiches and vegetable salads.

## COLLARDS

When the African slaves were brought over from their African homeland to the South to work on the plantations, they learned to make wholesome meals from the poorest ingredients, discarded scraps, and whatever foods they could grow for themselves. Since collards, along with the whole family of greens, grew profusely in the South, they became a popular item in many meals. They became a foundation of soul food, but haven't gotten the appreciation they deserve outside of the soul food venue.

Scraps such as pig's feet, ham hocks, brains, cow's testicles (also known as "mountain oysters"), and pig's intestines—better known as chitterlings or chitlins—that were discarded by plantation owners were used by slaves to season collards or other greens. Though these plantation workers had only a few vegetables and a limited number of rejected meat scraps to work with, they developed a knack for making them taste good. They fried, barbecued, and pickled these unedibles into delicacies.

As travelers arrived in the South from Europe and other parts of North America, they introduced new food items such as corn, rice, squash, and tomatoes. These, too, were incorporated into the greens and beans pot. A unique Southern cuisine was born. Slaves who worked in the plantation kitchens in the South contributed important nutritional balance to the simple Southern diet by serving collard greens at their masters' tables.

Collards are comprised of big, dark, oval green leaves with thick stems. They have a subtle taste somewhere between cabbage and kale. Both collards and kale are actually loose-leafed, non-heading wild cabbages that are ancestors of head cabbage. The major differences between collards and kale are the leaf shape, length of the stem, color, and flavor. While collards have a medium green color, smooth texture, and oval shape, most kale has dark, grayish-green, broad, crinkled leaves. On the flavor scale, collards are several degrees milder than kale. Initially, only the stems of the wild cabbages were eaten. (Even broccoli, in the beginning, was mainly cultivated for its calcium-rich stems.)

The vitamins and minerals in collard greens are more bioavailable when cooking breaks down the cell walls in the leaves. Although raw collards are definitely nutritious, this vegetable is preferable in its cooked state. Cooking this vegetable quadruples its bioavailable protein content per cup, and vitamin C availability triples. The B vitamins, calcium, iron, potassium, and zinc in collards are also more easily absorbed from cooked collards.

# WATERCRESS

Watercress is another leafy member of the cruciferous vegetable family. According to the Web site www.watercress.com (yes—it does exist!), watercress is the most ancient leafy green vegetable on record, having been consumed by ancient Persians, Greeks, and Romans. The site claims that the Greeks believed that watercress "could cure a deranged mind." It has historic uses as a breath freshener and palate cleanser.

Pliny the Elder, who lived from 23 to 79 A.D., listed over 40 medicinal uses for watercress, and included the belief that the smell of watercress would drive away snakes and neutralize scorpion venom! A Persian tradition was to feed it to their children to increase strength and stature. Its relative, arugula, is similarly peppery and flavorful.

While watercress isn't likely to replace antidepressants or mouthwash any time soon, it does contain natural phytochemicals—the sulforaphane group—that stimulate cell defenses against carcinogens. But watercress is particularly potent because of its high concentration of these natural compounds. In addition, the mustard oil present in the leaves and stem has antibiotic and anti-inflammatory properties. The main chemical that gives watercress its peppery flavor is *phenylethyl isothiocyanate*, or PEITC. This potent inhibitor of cancer development kills cancer cells and stimulates the detoxification of carcinogens in the body.

Like other bitter greens, watercress promotes good digestion. Gram for gram, watercress also has as much vitamin C as oranges and more calcium than milk, and is rich in folate besides. Eating watercress leaves daily is said to relieve migraines in some people. It is also brimming with beta- carotene— great for healthy skin and eyes.

With only 22 calories per 100-gram serving, you can eat all you want. Just be sure to rinse it well (at least three times with a little vinegar), especially if eating it raw. In France, potato and watercress soup—*potage cressionniere*—is a popular dish; in the UK, watercress sandwiches are a main- stay of afternoon tea. Is it coincidence that recent research found that residents of Britain and France are, overall, significantly healthier than Americans? There's more to it than watercress... probably.

Watercress has such a wide range of vitamins, minerals and trace elements that it is good for a great many conditions and should be present in your diet on a regular basis. Next to seaweed, it's the best source of iodine—a mineral essential for proper thyroid function.

Watercress contains more sulfur than any other vegetable except horseradish. Sulfur-rich foods play an important role in protein absorption, blood purifying, cell building, and maintaining healthy hair and skin. The potassium content of watercress gives it a diuretic action that draws excess fluid out of the body.

Chewing watercress is a folk remedy for bleeding gums. Fresh watercress juice, applied to the face and skin, is said to fade freckles, spots and blotches, and clear acne, blemishes, pimples, and blackheads. The juice can be applied at night and washed off in the morning. (You will need an extraction juicer to make juices from leafy greens; these juicers can cost between $200 and $600, but they are an excellent investment in your health. I recommend the Green Power Juicer, made by a company called Green Star.)

A natural beauty lotion can be made by mixing a tablespoon of honey with four tablespoons of watercress juice. Bottled and kept refrigerated, this lotion can be dabbed on the skin with cotton morning and evening (careful to avoid the eyes!) to bring out skin's natural beauty.

Watercress is a great source of the trace element *germanium*, which has antiviral, detoxifying, and antibiotic properties. Germanium helps to oxygenate the body, strengthens the bones and immune system, and fosters better intercellular communication. This little-known trace element also acts as an adaptogen, helping the body to achieve its healthiest possible balance. According to Monash Medical Centre's leading research nutritionist, watercress is one of a number of foods—including green tea and soy—that could interrupt one of the key pathways of developing lung, breast and bowel cancer.

Watercress stimulates digestive juices. The leaves are tangy-tasting and have a pungent, refreshing smell. The very best way to get the full nutritional value of watercress is to pick it just before eating. Add it to cooked dishes, salads, soups, stews, and stir-fries. It should not be cooked, but added to hot dishes right before they are served. Watercress, tomato and cheese make a great salad or sandwich combination. Try serving sprigs of watercress as a garnish on veggie platters. Try using it instead of basil when making pesto. Use the leaves in omelets, pies, quiche, casseroles, dips, rice dishes and stuffing.

# SPINACH

Spinach was first cultivated by the Persians; now, it's grown throughout the world. It was first used for its medicinal properties as a mild laxative, which are believed to be due to its rich content of *oxalic acid*—a nutrient that gives spinach its lemony flavor.

Although much lauded as a highly nutritious vegetable, spinach has one drawback. Although it contains high levels of iron and calcium, oxalic acid binds with these minerals and makes them almost completely unavailable for absorption in the GI tract. That gritty feeling you get on your teeth when eating raw spinach is the sensation of chewing on precipitated oxalic acid and calcium.

In health foodie circles, there is intense disagreement over whether spinach should be consumed raw or cooked. Some experts insist that spinach should only be eaten cooked; others, that it should never be cooked. The answer here—as is usually the case with such extremes in opinion—is that both sides are right. Cooking only reduces oxalate content slightly, about 5 to 15 percent; it doesn't make much difference in the availability of minerals to cook the life out of those emerald-green leaves. Cooking can increase the bioavailability of some of spinach's nutrients, but then you lose the life force of the enzymes that fresh spinach contains. You're best off eating *lots* of organic spinach; eat some of it raw, some of it cooked.

Spinach's reputation as a great source of iron was established based on faulty information—actually, due to a misplaced decimal point in research figures! Spinach is, however, extraordinarily high in vitamin C and rich in the B vitamin riboflavin. It has a very high chlorophyll content, plus plenty of carotenes, folate, magnesium, potassium, and vitamins E, $B_1$, and $B_6$. Research has shown that people who eat spinach regularly are less likely to develop lung cancer.

## SPINACH EXTRACT SHOWS PROMISE AS NATURAL APPETITE SUPPRESSANT

A class of substances called *thylakoids* has been isolated from the membranes of chloroplasts, the organelles within plant cells that contain chlorophyll. Thylakoids appear to be good sources of minerals, amino acids, and essential fatty acids; they have also been found to inhibit the digestion of fat. The end result: a slowing-down of fat digestion and increased signals of satiety (fullness) going to the brain.

Swedish husband-and-wife research team Per-Ake Albertsson and Charlotte Erlanson-Albertsson—one, a biochemistry professor who studies photosynthesis, and the other an obesity and appetite control researcher—decided to use spinach as their source of thylakoids. In test-tube studies, they found that fat was broken down more slowly in the presence of thylakoids; and then, they discovered that administering thylakoids to lab animals fed a high-fat diet suppresses their appetites and helps them to lose weight. The animals' blood lipid levels decreased as well.

The research team makes clear that thylakoids, if ever isolated into supplement form, would have to be taken with a meal. This phytochemical has to be consumed with fats (lipids) to serve the purpose of appetite suppression. Thylakoids are believed to slow fat digestion by surrounding fat molecules with a coating that blocks the action of pancreatic lipase, the enzyme that breaks down fats in the digestive system.

To get the appetite-suppressant benefits of spinach from eating the food itself, it's estimated that you would have to consume about half a kilogram—that's about a pound—of spinach per day. I think it's doable, but you might tire of spinach rather quickly on that kind of regimen. Researchers are working to isolate thylakoids and concentrate them into a dietary supplement that could be added to foods that are rich in fat, like pies or cookies.

Like other leafy greens, spinach has a high water content; when cooked, it shrinks considerably. One pound of leaves reduces to about one cup cooked.

Spinach is another vegetable that has a different nutritional profile cooked than raw—it releases more of its iron and calcium when cooked. It's best to include it in both forms in your diet:

- Lightly steamed spinach with butter is a great side dish. The water left over after cooking is rich in iron and other water-soluble nutrients; save the cooking water for soups or drink it.

- If you've invested in a juice extractor, try some spinach juice. It is said to be the most potent vegetable juice when it comes to the prevention of cancer cell formation. Combine spinach with carrot, apple, and ginger for a refreshing A.M. cocktail.

- Use baby spinach leaves in salads, or use them instead of lettuce. Try spinach, mandarin orange slices, and almond slices tossed in a little bit of rice vinegar.

- Stir raw spinach into soups, scrambled eggs, or pasta sauces right before serving.

According to the Environmental Working Group, spinach is a highly pesticide-intensive crop. Choose organic spinach to avoid taking in toxic pesticides.

## SWISS CHARD

This leafy green is a member of the same family as spinach and beets. Its flavor is bitter like beet greens, but slightly reminiscent of spinach in its saltiness. It boasts an impressive list of health-promoting nutrients. A single cup of cooked Swiss chard supplies nearly one-third of your daily potassium requirement—something to consider if you are hypertensive. (Adequate potassium intake can help reduce blood pressure naturally.) Swiss chard is packed with minerals, and is an excellent source of vitamins C, K, and E, along with a full complement of carotenes and other antioxidants. Eating chard regularly promotes the health of the eyes, cardiovascular system, and immune system.

Chard is hardier than spinach, and requires slightly longer cooking times. Prepare it like kale: two tablespoons each of olive oil and water; add garlic to the oil first, then the water and chard; remove the center ribs of the leaves if you like, but you don't need to; cover and cook at medium heat until wilted. Chard is good in pasta sauces, soups, and egg dishes.

# BEET GREENS

It's too bad that most beet-eaters toss the leaves and eat the sweet roots alone. These greens are a great source of vitamins, minerals, trace elements and amino acids. The greens of beet plants are actually much better for you nutritionally than the beet itself; they have blood-cleansing qualities and taste great when prepared right. Try a beet salad made with steamed beets (steam for about 30 minutes, at which point their skins slip off easily), chopped into bite-sized pieces, and lightly steamed or boiled chopped beet leaves. Mix with a dijon vinaigrette and some toasted pumpkin seeds.

## GREENS: AN AYURVEDIC PERSPECTIVE

As Ayurvedic physician Vasant Lad says, "Bitter is better"—especially when it comes to detoxifying the body. If you were to visit an Ayurvedic physician who found your diet to be too heavy and sweet—like the typical Western diet almost always is—he would likely recommend that you counteract that heavy sweetness with more bitter, dark, leafy greens.

Next time you crave sweets, go for something bitter and leafy and green, instead. A vegetable juice made from leafy greens will knock out your sweet craving before you can say "ice cold milk and an Oreo cookie."

Light, pungent, and rich in vitamins and minerals, dark leafy vegetables like kale, collards, watercress, beet greens, chard, arugula, dandelion, chicory, mustard and turnip greens are all described in Ayurveda as specific healers for the liver and immune system.

Most greens have a pungent vipak (digestive effect), which is why Ayurvedic doctors recommend that they be prepared with generous amounts of cooling coriander powder. Small amounts are well-tolerated by most constitutions (an exception: those with strong Pitta or Vata constitutions shouldn't eat too much spinach, arugula, or Swiss chard, all of which are high in oxalic acid), and are useful medicinally in the treatment of lung and liver disorders.

Source: *The Ayurvedic Cookbook* by Amanda Morningstar

Juiced, beet greens add color and blood-cleansing strength to your vegetable juice cocktail. Be sure to mix beet green juice with other vegetable or fruit juices; the intense cleansing effects of beet green juice can bring on some unpleasant reactions if you drink too much at one time. Young beet leaves add a streak of color and a delightful taste to any salad. More mature leaves can be used in soups, dropped briefly in boiling water, or steamed until tender.

Beet greens have traditionally been used as a natural remedy for anemia, circulatory problems, kidney, liver and bladder problems, skin problems, eye fatigue, menopause, and general tiredness, and to improve the circulation of lymph (the fluid that carries immune cells around the body and helps to eliminate waste and toxins from the circulatory system).

## SPROUTS

Wanted! A vegetable that will:

- Grow in any climate

- Rival meat in nutritive value

- Mature in three to five days

- Thrive regardless of season

- Require neither soil nor sunshine

- Rival tomatoes in vitamin C content

- Be free of waste in preparation

- Require no cooking or other preparation once grown

During World War II, all these criteria were listed by Clive M. McKay, Ph.D., a professor of nutrition at Cornell University, who was researching the amazing health-promoting properties of sprouted soybeans. Since then, we've learned that sprouts made from all sorts of legumes, nuts, and seeds will create perfect little nutritional powerhouses, loaded with living energy, enzymes, fiber, vitamins, and minerals.

Medicinally and nutritionally, sprouts go way back. Ancient Chinese physicians prescribed sprouts for curing many disorders over 5,000 years ago. Sprouts continue to be a staple in the diets of Asian-Americans. Although accounts of sprouting appear in the Bible in the Book of Daniel, it took centuries for the West to fully realize their value. Today, raw-foods proponents make use of sprouting to lend variety to their diets of vegetables, fruits, nuts, and seeds. Sprouted seeds and beans are used to make dehydrated crackers and breads, seed "cheeses," and other delicious foods. During World War II, considerable interest in sprouts was sparked in the United States by Dr. McKay and his team of researchers. They and other researchers at the universities of Pennsylvania, Minnesota, McGill, and Yale found that sprouts retain the B-complex vitamins present in the original seed, and show a dramatic 300 percent increase in carotenes and a 500 percent increase in vitamin C content over what is present in the unsprouted seed.

During the sprouting process, starches are converted to simple sugars, making sprouts easy to digest. They are full of potential energy, preparing to transform from seed to growing plant, and their enzymes are working at a fever pitch. When you eat sprouts, those enzymes promote better digestion and enhance your energy levels.

The National Cancer Institute and the National Institutes of Health both recommend eating five fresh fruits and vegetables every day. A great way to help reach that goal is to include sprouts. Just toss them onto whatever you're eating, or munch them on their own.

Buckwheat sprouts have more chlorophyll than spinach, kale, cabbage or parsley. Alfalfa, sunflower, clover and radish sprouts are all 4 percent protein; soybean sprouts are 28 percent protein, while lentil and pea sprouts are 26 percent protein. Think of it this way: Sprouted peas contain twice the protein of eggs and only one-tenth the fat!

Spicy radish sprouts are very high in vitamin C and carotenes—and contain 10 times more calcium than a potato. These little vitamin factories contain 39 times the beta-carotene of a mature radish. Sprout lovers have been heard to say that they can feel the vitamins when eating these tiny phytochemical factories.

Alfalfa, radish, broccoli, clover and soybean sprouts, in particular, contain concentrated amounts of phytochemicals (plant compounds) that can protect us against disease. Plant estrogens (phytoestrogens) in these sprouts function as "weak" estrogens that occupy estrogen receptors on cells in the body, blocking the carcinogenic, proliferative effects of environmental xenoestrogens (toxic chemicals that act like crazy killer estrogens in the body). Many women, as they near menopause, stop making adequate progesterone—estrogen's natural balancer in the body—and end up with too much of their own natural estrogens, resulting in painful, difficult periods, weight gain, mood swings, and even fibroids in the uterus. Eating sprouts rich in phytoestrogens can help reduce the intensity of this estrogen-overloaded state in women going through this stage of life.

Phytoestrogens have been found to increase bone formation and density and prevent bone breakdown that leads to osteoporosis. They are also helpful in controlling hot flashes, menopause, PMS, and fibrocystic breasts tumors.

Broccoli's good, but broccoli sprouts might be even better. Johns Hopkins University School of Medicine researchers found substantial amounts of glucosinolates and isothiocyanates in broccoli sprouts. These potent inducers of Phase II liver detoxification enzymes help to protect cells against malignant transformation. Broccoli sprouts contain 10 to 100 times greater concentrations of these enzymes than mature broccoli plants.

Alfalfa sprouts are one of our finest food sources of saponins, which help to lower "bad" LDL cholesterol and triglycerides, without affecting levels of "good" HDL cholesterol. Saponins stimulate the immune system by increasing the activity of natural killer cells, including T- lymphocytes and interferon—both major defenses against cancer and infection.

Sprouts also contain an abundance of highly active antioxidants that protect DNA and slow the aging process. It makes sense that sprouts would act as a sort of "fountain of youth"—after all, they're a perfect representation of the miracle of birth. The sprouting process is where a lifeless seed becomes a plant!

Legumes (beans) contain a few substances which, if eaten in too-great quantities, may cause some digestive unpleasantness, including intestinal gas. Even sprouted legumes can have this effect, but sprouting and rinsing seems to greatly reduce these digestive inhibitors. If you find that they do cause you to become a bit gassier than you'd like, simply eat them in smaller amounts, or cook your sprouted legumes as you would any other bean to further improve their digestibility. Although the enzymes will be denatured by the heat, sprouted legumes are still far richer in vitamins, minerals, and other nutrients than unsprouted legumes.

## AKTIVATED BARLEY: AN ANCIENT PRE-SPROUTED BARLEY DEVELOPED BY THE GREEKS AND ROMANS

Perhaps you've heard that grain products such as barley and oatmeal lower "bad" LDL cholesterol, as well as the risk of heart disease and diabetes. This is due in large part to their content of *beta-glucans*, the ultimate "good carbohydrate." Aktivated Barley was developed based on techniques used in ancient Greece and Rome to transform barley into a highly nutritious food for athletes, and for infants whose mothers could not breastfeed them. You can think of it as "pre-sprouted" barley—the sprouting process has been activated, but the sprout has not yet formed when the grain is consumed. This food is an extraordinarily rich source of beta-glucan and other nutrients that can support optimal cardiovascular health, blood sugar balance, and athletic performance.

Aktivated Barley is used by United Nations workers to help ease the tragedy of famine in impoverished or war-torn parts of the world. Discovering this ancient food and participating in efforts to make it available to people in need has been one of the most rewarding aspects of my work. Only two servings a day of Aktivated Barley can provide hungry people with long-lasting energy, comprehensive nutrition, and endurance. When used along with concentrated green foods made from algaes and cereal grasses, this supplement can provide unparalleled nutrition to people who desperately need it.

Ancient Greeks and Romans soaked barley for 24 hours, mashed it into gruel, then boiled it, which barely initiates the sprouting process. The resulting mixture is strained, preserving the nutrient-rich liquid. This is a process similar to the one used to make a raw food called Rejuvelac, which was developed by Ann Wigmore. Rejuvelac is a staple of the living food diet offered at the Hippocrates Health Institute's centers and in programs like it all over the world. It is used to make Ann's famous Energy Soup—one of the most healing foods known to humankind. More on this shortly.

The modern process is more high-tech, using pressure instead of heat to activate enzymes and yield high concentrations of beta-glucans.

## MAKE YOUR OWN SPROUTS

Making sprouts is easy. All you need is a colander and some organic sprouting seeds, legumes, grains, or nuts. Rinse the seeds thoroughly; soak the seeds in water for 12 hours; then place them in a colander, sprouting jar, or other sprouting vessel and rinse them twice a day. Allow them to drain in a cool, dry place, out of the sun. In a few days you'll have sprouts! For more detailed instruction and tips on seeds and equipment, check out the book by Steve Meyerowitz, *Sprouts: The Miracle Food* (Sproutman Publications, 1998), or *The Sprouting Book* by Ann Wigmore (Avery, 1986; a classic!), both available at Amazon.com and at many health food stores.

## ANN WIGMORE'S ENERGY SOUP

Can a single recipe save lives? According to the testimonials of many who have discovered the recipe for Ann Wigmore's Energy Soup, the answer to this question is yes. People with all kinds of illnesses, malnourished people, individuals with uncontrollable cravings and addictions have all found an answer with the regular consumption of this plant-based concoction.

Energy Soup is a cornerstone of the living foods diet. It is a blended mixture of greens, other vegetables, sprouts, Rejuvelac (the liquid strained from fermented grains), and dulse, a tasty type of sea vegetable. The recipe goes something like this:

- Base of Rejuvelac, water, or unpasteurized apple juice

- Five cups of home-grown or store-bought organic baby greens

- One to two cups of bean sprouts

- One-half to one avocado

- One apple

- Two tablespoons of seaweed (dulse, kelp, or nori)

- Optional additional ingredients: a clove of garlic, some extra greens, a banana, extra apple or apple juice concentrate, soaked sunflower seeds or raw nuts, watermelon, raw honey, brown rice syrup...Ann encouraged her students to experiment to find a mixture that agreed with their palates.

Simply toss all ingredients into a high-powered blender or food-processor. Add as much liquid as you need to add to make it soup-like and to achieve the thickness you prefer.

Rejuvelac is a fermented beverage made at home with organic grains. It is rich in protein, carbohydrates, and *Lactobacilli* (friendly bacteria). Make it in a two-quart mason jar. Boil the jar for three to five minutes and cool before adding two cups of cereal grains, such as rye, barley, wheat, millet, triticale, spelt, or amaranth. Rinse the grain until water runs clear, then add enough water to nearly fill the jar. Let soak for 12 hours to begin the sprouting process. Then, turn the jar over to allow water to drain. Keep the jar in a warm place (68 to 80 degrees) and rinse two to six times over the next 24 to 72 hours, keeping the grains moist but not wet. Small sprouts will start to be seen coming from the seeds.

Once the grain has been sprouted, fermentation is next. Simply fill the two-quart jar (with the grain inside it) to the top with water. Put the sprouting lid on and let it sit for 24 to 72 hours at 68 to 80 degrees. Low light is fine, but avoid direct sunlight. Once it's ready, the Rejuvelac will smell pleasant and have a lemony flavor.

Place a cone-shaped permanent coffee filter or other type of fine-mesh filter over the mouth of a jar, then strain the liquid off of the grains. This liquid is the Rejuvelac. (Cook the sprouted grains as cereal or a grain side dish, or use them to make dehydrated crackers or bread.) Rejuvelac will keep a few days—up to one week—in the refrigerator. It should taste sour, but not foul.

You can use Rejuvelac in Energy Soup, or drink it plain. It's an acquired taste, but as superfoods go, this one is tops. More information can be found in Ann Wigmore's books, *The Blending Book* and *Recipes for Long Life*.

# *Chapter Seven*

## SEA VEGETABLE SALAD

For several years you couldn't open a book or magazine about healthful eating and not see a story extolling the amazing benefits of soy. Over and over again, the same line was spun, with slight variations: "Asians have much lower risk of breast cancer and osteoporosis than Americans do, and they eat a lot more soy than Americans!" The message, of course, is that soy is the big Asian health secret to long life and good health.

Let's get real. Soy does have some benefits (when fermented, organic, and sprouted), but it also has a long list of potential negatives, which I'm not going to bring up here. Soy or non-soy is only one tiny difference between the Asian and typical American diet. Besides, it turns out that Asians don't really eat that much more soy than Americans do; a study of about 5,000 Japanese men and women found that daily soy intake was equivalent to about a half-cup of tofu or an eight-ounce cup of soymilk. I know some Americans who guzzle soymilk three times a day and eat tofu two or three times a week!

Asians eat far more vegetables and seafood than Americans do. There are also drastic differences in lifestyle, spiritual practices, medical practices and philosophies, and activity levels. Reducing the longevity and good health of

Asians to their consumption of soy is like reducing Americans' obesity and chronic disease to their consumption of a single food...say, french fries. It just isn't that simple.

Here's one example of the difference between massive generalizations and the much more nuanced picture of reality: Did you know that most Asian dishes that contain tofu or other soy foods also contain sea vegetables? Americans don't eat these mineral-rich, fiber-rich, nutrient-dense vegetables nearly as often as Asians do. One might guess that sea vegetables are, in fact, the big secret to lifelong health, the Asian way. In fact, the average traditional Asian diet contains a whopping 25 times more sea vegetables than the average traditional American diet. Coincidence? I think not!

We can't boil down the differences in Asian and American diets to one food—but by the time you finish this chapter, I hope to open your mind to the strong possibility that these exotic vegetables from the sea could well make a significant contribution to the good health of Asians who stick with their traditional diet.

You would expect to be served sea vegetables in an Asian restaurant: seaweed salads, miso soup made with dulse, and nori-wrapped sushi where Japanese cuisine is served, or a stir-fry of tofu and hijiki in a Chinese restaurant, for example. But you might not have known that sea vegetables are used in traditional cuisines all around the world—particularly those of people who have long lived right next to the ocean. In the British Isles, for example, a fried breakfast bread is made with rolled oats and a strain of nori seaweed called *laver*. Traditional foods from Scandinavia, Scotland, Ireland, Iceland, New Zealand, Australia, and the Pacific Islands all incorporate sea vegetables.

Sea vegetables and freshwater plants are extremely rich sources of highly bioavailable nutrition. Not all of them are green in color—giant kelp, for instance, is dusky brown, and *Lithothamnium calcareum* is purplish-whitish—but they are photosynthetic plants that use chlorophyll to make sugars from the light of the sun, so they deserve to be included here in *The Green Foods Bible*.

In this chapter, I'll tell you about some of my favorite sea vegetables, and about the benefits they can have in a well-rounded plant-based nutrition program. You'll learn more about kelp, and about dulse and a lesser-known freshwater plant called *Hydrilla verticillata*. I'll round out the discussion with some information on a sea plant called *Lithothamnium calcareum*, which happens to be one of nature's most abundant sources of highly bioavailable calcium. I'll also give you some handy tips for using commonly available sea vegetables like nori, hijiki, and wakame in your home cooking.

Sea vegetables differ from greens that grow on land in their high mineral density and relatively high protein content. Most sea vegetables are rich in important minerals like calcium, magnesium, and iron. Their mineral composition mirrors that of seawater, which, in turn, mirrors the mineral composition of our own bodies—which are really just big packets of seawater that can stand up and walk around.

Bathing in the salty ocean is rejuvenative and healing. Eating sea vegetables is a way to bring that rejuvenative power inside your body. Using sea vegetables topically—in skin care products, body wraps, and shampoos, for example—helps us to feel a little of that wonderful just-bathed-in-the-sea feeling every day.

## A SEAWEED STORY

All along the Pacific coast of North America, you can find enormous colonies of giant kelp. Individual plants can grow at a rate of 12 inches per day, reaching heights of 100 or more feet—another example of a plant that is so perfectly adapted to thrive that it has existed unchanged for millions, even billions of years. Like the microalgaes, kelp's ability to rapidly grow and proliferate makes it an excellent candidate for helping to reduce world-wide hunger and malnutrition. Giant kelp is at the base of a marine food chain that is essential for the survival of the marine food web overall.

There are some 800 species of kelp in the world. These plants are anchored to rocks on the sea floor by a "holdfast," which looks like a root system but isn't. Giant kelp are actually classified as a type of giant algae— which, among other things, means that it doesn't have a root system. That's right— microalgae like chlorella and spirulina are in the same plant family as giant kelp! The other edible seaweeds, including dulse, arame, wakame, nori, and hijiki, are also considered to be types of algae.

Kelp requires plenty of light, so it has to grow in relatively shallow water. Giant kelp's long, hollow stems branch into large, flat leaves. At the base of each leaf is a small bladder that holds air, lending the plant plenty of buoyancy as it grows towards the water's surface. It grows in clusters that form kelp forests, which are known to be one of the richest wildlife habitats anywhere in the ocean. Snails, otters, many breeds of fish and sea birds, anemones, abalone, sea urchins, dolphins, and other animals spend their lives in and around kelp forests. The plant has male parts, which fertilize its female parts to make new kelp spores. New spores drift to the bottom of the ocean to grow into yet another swaying brown frond of kelp. As the fronds reach the water's surface, they continue to grow, forming a canopy.

If you've never had the opportunity to snorkel or scuba dive in a kelp forest, it's something you really ought to put on your list. Down in the depths, you can look up and see the giant kelp stems gently undulating with the move-ment of the currents and the waves. You have to be careful, though, not to get entangled in the long stems, especially where they form a canopy. You've got to wait for a clearing, then descend into what a PBS program for kids aptly called "the cathedral of the sea." If you have to cross a canopy of kelp on top of the water, trying to swim through it will get you tangled; you're better off crawling right on top of the buoyant leaves.

One of the best spots for kelp exploration is in the Monterey Canyon, a 70-mile-long stretch of ocean off of Monterey in central California. This ecosystem is unbelievably rich, and on any given day you can stand on the shore and see sea otters, sea lions, harbor seals, and even gray whales. Four hundred species of fish and 25 species of marine mammals thrive there. The Monterey Bay Aquarium, built in an old Cannery Row sardine-packing plant, is well worth a visit, too; it contains a Kelp Forest exhibit, 66 feet long and 28 feet deep. Inside, you can see thousands of glittery silver sardines darting to and fro among the kelp stems like a single body.

Dive instructors will tell you that if you ever do get entangled in strands of kelp, you can bite the strands into pieces to free yourself. Kelp is not only edible, it happens to be one of the more nourishing foods you can eat. (Most authorities recommend you avoid harvesting your own, however, because periodically it may form toxins that can give you serious gastrointestinal difficulty.) Giant kelp and other sea vegetables are harvested on a large scale to make additives for processed foods. Derivatives of seaweed are found in salad dressings, cakes, ice cream, and beverages.

## KELP RISKS: TOO MUCH IODINE?

It is possible to get too much iodine with kelp supplements or by eating a lot of kelp. Although iodine deficiency afflicts millions of people worldwide—damaging thyroid health and causing irreversible developmental disabilities, including mental retardation, in the babies of women who are iodine-deficient—iodine deficiency is extremely rare in developed nations, where iodized salt is pretty much the only kind used.

A ¼ cup serving of kelp contains 277 percent of the daily RDA of iodine, which is 150 mcg (micrograms) per day (unless you're pregnant—then, it's 220 mcg; or breastfeeding—then, it's 290 mcg). One European study of kelp supplements found that the pills contained anywhere from 17 mcg to 57,000 mcg (57 milligrams) per dose!

According to the National Academy of Sciences, the safe upper limit for daily iodine intake is 1.1 milligrams; that's about seven times the minimum you should take in each day. Taking dramatically more than the recommended daily maximum each day can cause hyperthyroidism, where the thyroid gland becomes overactive, raising metabolic rate, heart rate, and blood pressure beyond safe limits. Too much iodine can also worsen acne.

If you are inspired to use a kelp supplement, use one from a reputable company—ask a trusted advisor at your health food store, or your natural health practitioner. The amount of iodine in the supplement should be labeled on the bottle, and you should be able to verify that the measurement is accurate with the manufacturer.

Another potential hazard that has (very rarely) cropped up with the use of kelp: arsenic poisoning. In two case studies, people who had been using kelp regularly as a supplement were found to have arsenic poisoning; their illnesses were traced back to high arsenic content in the supplements. This plant can accumulate arsenic from ocean water. If you choose to use a kelp supplement, make sure it is from a reputable manufacturer like Platinum that assures its product has been tested and contains none of this chemical.

On the brighter side, sea vegetables like kelp do not contain appreciable amounts of carcinogenic, immune-system-damaging, fat-soluble toxins commonly found in fish and shellfish, including PCBs and dioxins.

Scientists in Great Britain, who are just as concerned over the epidemics of obesity and colon cancer as we are in the U.S., have recommended that *alginates*—a high-fiber, very low-fat component of seaweed that is already widely added to processed foods as a stabilizer and water retainer—be added to junk food, bread, and burgers to reduce fat and dramatically enhance fiber and nutrient content. Alginates are soothing and healing to the intestinal tract and help to promote *peristalsis*—the muscular contractions that propel food through the GI tract during the digestive process.

Test-tube and animal studies show kelp's promise as a natural preventative against influenza, herpes, and HIV infections. Like red marine algae, kelp appears to have the kind of antiviral effects that have long eluded those who would love to make a truly safe, effective antiviral pharmaceutical drug.

One 1/4-cup serving of kelp contains 10 percent of the recommended daily intake of folate and about 8 percent of the DV for magnesium. It is nature's richest source of the mineral iodine, which is crucial for proper thyroid gland function. Like all the other sea vegetables, it contains abundant fiber and some vitamin $B_{12}$ (the jury's still out as to whether it's bioavailable; for now, don't rely on sea vegetables to get your vitamin $B_{12}$).

Kelp has been billed as a weight-loss aid—probably due to the fact that it can increase the activity of the thyroid, the gland that acts as primary driver of metabolic rate. If your thyroid begins to crank out more of its hormones, you'll burn more calories, your heart will speed up, your blood pressure will rise, and you'll feel more energy, probably in the form of jitteriness. While this might sound like a good thing for someone who wants to lose weight, creating a hyper-thyroid state actually can end up being quite dangerous. This is not a safe weight-loss strategy.

There is substantial overlap among the sea vegetables in terms of their nutritional composition and health benefits. We've taken a close look at kelp, one of the better researched sea vegetables; now, let's widen our lens and look at the health benefits of sea vegetables as a green food "group."

## RESEARCH DEMONSTRATES HEALTH BENEFITS OF EDIBLE SEAWEEDS

Some of the more promising research on kelp and the other sea vegetables has revealed potential uses for the prevention of cancer—most notably, breast and intestinal cancers. So far, the studies have primarily been done in test tubes and on lab animals, but the evidence that comes from this research seems adequate to push forward into human studies.

Sea vegetables in general have been studied intently for their health-promoting properties. The National Cancer Institute and other highly esteemed institutions are studying ocean plants' anti-inflammatory, antiviral, antimicrobial, antifungal, and anti-cancer effects.

Seaweeds are roughly categorized as red, brown, or green, and although there are hundreds of species, only a few are commonly eaten by humans: arame, hijiki, nori, wakame, dulse, and kelp. Many others are used medicinally, but they all share similar benefits.

These foods are packed with minerals and B vitamins (particularly folate, pantothenic acid, and riboflavin)—nutrients that collaborate to support the health and proper function of the adrenal glands, which are our first responders in times of stress. The adrenals produce "fight-or-flight" hormones and other longer-acting hormones that are required for us to cope with and rise to the various challenges we face. Making sea vegetables a regular part of your diet will help you maintain good adrenal function.

Sea vegetables are also highly alkaline, helping to counter the acidity of the typical Western diet.

## SEAWEEDS VS. CANCER

Overall, scientists who research breast cancer are in agreement that sea vegetables are protective against this disease. Much evidence suggests that this protective effect has something to do with seaweeds' stores of iodine and selenium and their effects on the thyroid gland. Research is ongoing, but at this point, the evidence is strong enough that I would highly recommend that all women concerned about breast cancer should integrate sea veggies into their diets—*today*.

Seaweeds have general anti-cancer actions, and are especially promising against breast, cervical, and gastrointestinal cancers. Aside from the iodine/selenium content, sea vegetables are promising cancer fighters because:

- They have potent antioxidant activity.

- They have proven anti-angiogenic and anti-proliferative effects in test tube and animal studies of breast, skin, and cervical cancer.

- The fiber in sea vegetables is particularly good at binding to and removing carcinogenic toxins from the body.

- They are rich in *polyphenols*, nutrients with known cancer-slowing activity.

- Rats fed kelp along with a breast carcinogen called DMBA were better able to increase antioxidant production in their livers, and the expected oxidative damage in the animals' livers did not occur after DMBA administration.

- Seaweeds contain *phytoestrogens* in the form of *lignans*. Phytoestrogens are weakly estrogenic substances found in plants that can block the cancer-accelerating effects of xenoestrogens (synthetic chemicals), and even the body's own estrogens when too many are produced relative to their balancing hormone, progesterone. (This, according to hormone expert John Lee, M.D., and others, often happens in the years preceding menopause). When kelp was administered to female rats, their normal menstrual cycle was lengthened—a longer cycle is better when it comes to cancer prevention. When added to human ovarian cells, the kelp extract increased production of progesterone, which is believed to aid in balancing estrogen's proliferative (cancer-accelerating) effects. Binding of estradiol, the most proliferative form of estrogen produced in the body, was reduced with kelp supplementation. The authors of the study, a group at the University of California at Berkeley School of Public Health, conclude that "dietary kelp may contribute to the lower incidence of hormone-dependent cancers among the Japanese."

- An earlier paper by the same research group at Berkeley found that three women who took a kelp supplement—this one was *Fucus vesiculosus*, also known as bladder wrack—had significant increases in the length of their menstrual cycles. Estrogen levels were reduced and progesterone levels enhanced in these women.

- Both men and women produce estrogens in fat cells. The more fat a person carries, the more estrogen their bodies probably contain. This may contribute powerfully to the known increase in cancer in people who are obese. Lignans reduce this production of extra estrogens in fat cells.

- Test tube studies have also found that lignans reduce *angiogenesis*, where cancerous tumors sprout their own blood vessel system in an effort to grow and spread. Dulse, hijiki, and arame are other sea vegetables rich in lignans.

• Another compound found in sea vegetables, *fucoidans*, has shown anti-proliferative effects on lymphoma cells; it also has been found to promote *apoptosis*—the selective death of cancerous cells.

## REMOVAL OF TOXINS

Experimental evidence suggests that seaweed—particularly brown kelp—binds with heavy metals such as mercury, lead, and aluminum in the body. Kelp is rich in *alginates*, a gel-like fiber that traps and removes toxins like metals through the gastrointestinal tract. Consuming sea vegetables has been found to prevent the absorption of heavy metals as you ingest them. This information suggests that people should consume seaweeds any time they consume tuna, which is known to have high mercury concentrations.

Powdered seaweed extracts are a promising high-fiber addition to processed foods. If added to bread, such an extract could quadruple its fiber content without changing its taste or texture.

## REDUCTION OF INFLAMMATION AND MUSCLE CONSTRICTION

Kelp and other seaweeds contain fucans, which are sulfated polysaccharides—a kind of complex carbohydrate. Fucans are remarkably effective natural anti-inflammatories, which makes sea vegetables a good choice for people with arthritis, allergies, asthma, or autoimmune diseases.

## NATURAL SKIN CARE FROM THE SEA

Research performed in France has demonstrated that algae micronutrients are readily absorbed through the skin. Any organic skin product, hair product, or cosmetic that includes appreciable amounts of seaweed is probably a good bet.

If you like to make your own, try this seaweed skin mask: Mix a table- spoon of kelp powder and a tablespoon of dulse powder with just enough warm water to make a mayonnaise-like paste. Smooth it onto your face; let it dry; then wash off. You can add a half-tablespoon of aloe vera gel for softening or a half-tablespoon of honey to help remove dead skin particles.

Sea vegetables also help to reduce muscle constriction by providing a source of bioavailable magnesium, a mineral with relaxant properties. Magnesium is found abundantly in a plant-based, unprocessed diet.

## SOME OTHER WATER PLANTS OF NOTE

I'd like to address two other water plants here that don't have culinary uses. So far, they are only useful when made into dietary supplements, but they jive quite well with my philosophy of using whole foods rich in specific nutrients as supplemental sources of those nutrients, rather than using isolated, single nutrients.

*Hydrilla verticillata.* This is a freshwater plant, like chlorella and spirulina. It's not an algae, but a macrophyte—a class of plants that includes mosses, ferns, liverworts, and other rooted plants. Hydrilla has a long stem, a deep root structure, many leaves, and a bright green hue.

It was introduced a while back as an aquarium plant, but it escaped into the wild—probably when someone dumped the contents of his fishbowl into a stream or lake. Hydrilla grows so well that it quickly became a plant pest, encroaching on natural plant ecosystems all over the nation. At a rate of an inch of growth per day, you can imagine how this aquatic weed could quickly stake its claim. The plants can reach a length of 25 feet or more.

When a plant can grow like this, it seems natural to explore its use as a food. It turns out hydrilla is packed with nutrients: carotenoids, chlorophyll, selenium, vitamin C (six times more than in oranges), gamma-linoleic acid (an essential fatty acid, excellent for the skin).

Hydrilla is a terrific source of beta-carotene, containing almost 20,000 IU in 10.5 grams of the plant. It is also rich in calcium, containing 13 or more percent calcium when dehydrated. A tablespoon of powdered, dehydrated hydrilla contains between 624 and 700 mg of elemental calcium, along with abundant potassium, vitamin $B_{12}$ (again, not sure whether it's reliable as your only source; don't rely on it alone) and iron. As if these qualities weren't enough to recommend it, hydrilla is also high in the amino acid lysine, which makes it a good preventative against herpes outbreaks.

*Lithothamnium calcareum.* This mouthful of a name describes an interesting type of algae. It's a calcareous algae, meaning that it looks more like coral than algae; reddish-violet and small, with branches only two to three millimeters long, *Lithothamnium* is found most abundantly in oceans off of Ireland and Scotland.

This algae has been sold in powdered form as a soil additive for years— in fact, many seaweeds have been used for this purpose, and they are excellent for replenishing mineral content in soil. What makes this particular plant special is its very high content of calcium. It is already used as a soy milk additive, supplying bioavailable, naturally complexed calcium. Supplement manufacturers are starting to catch on, using *Lithothamnium* to make natural calcium supplements.

## HOW TO ADD SEA VEGETABLES TO YOUR DIET

Although your intentions might be terrific, you may find yourself in a state of confusion once you are standing in front of the dried sea vegetable display at your local health food store. Some of its black and squiggly; some of its brown or green and leafy; and some is ironed into flat black sheets. What the heck are you supposed to do with this stuff, anyhow?

Good news to those of you who wrinkle your nose at the thought of consuming seaweed: These plants are high in glutamate, an amino acid that elicits the so-called "fifth taste," known as *umami*. Umami has been variously described as meaty, savory, and pungent. In other words, seaweed tastes good—especially if you know how to use it. Here are some suggestions for painlessly and enjoyably adding sea vegetables to your diet:

*Arame*—soak in warm water for 10 to 15 minutes, then simmer in rice wine (sake), tamari, and lemon juice for 20 minutes and serve sprinkled with sesame seeds.

*Dulse*—can be fried in sesame oil to make "dulse chips," which can be used as a replacement for bacon; or add raw to any soup or casserole that contains potatoes (the flavors and textures complement each other well); some people like to just eat it dried right out of the bag—it has a jerky-like texture and salty flavor; or snip it into tiny pieces with kitchen scissors and use it as a condiment to flavor salads, rice, or soup.

*Hijiki*—before using, soak in warm water for five minutes; then rinse, chop, and combine with sliced cucumber, rice vinegar, and a dash of sugar.

*Kelp*—use powdered kelp to replace salt as a seasoning; you can mix it with garlic powder and white pepper to enhance its flavor.

*Kombu*—add a four- to six-inch-long strip to cooking water when cooking beans to speed cooking time and reduce gassiness; add to soup broths and remove after soup is done cooking.

*Nori*—briefly toast sheets over a flame or electric burner until they turn deep, emerald green; eat plain or use to wrap rice and vegetables (add some rice vinegar to the rice first to make it sticky), then slice into rounds with a very sharp knife; wrap tuna or salmon salad in nori instead of making them into sandwiches.

*Wakame*—the seaweed used traditionally to flavor miso soup; can also be used in rice—here's a recipe from the George Mateljan Foundation Web site, www.whfoods.com: rinse and soak wakame in 2 ½ cups of warm water for five minutes, then squeeze out the water and reserve for cooking the rice; chop the seaweed, and combine with sautéed chopped dulse, onion, and garlic; add one cup of long-grain brown rice and the soaking water; cover and cook at low heat for 35 minutes, until all the water is absorbed.

For more on cooking with sea vegetables, check out the Web site of the Mendocino Sea Vegetable Company, www.seaweed.net. At their site, you can buy their cookbook or a wide variety of sea vegetables. Or, buy the wonderful cookbook authored by macrobiotic chef and cooking instructor, Jill Gusman, *Vegetables from the Sea: Everyday Cooking with Sea Greens*. It's available at Amazon. com. Sea vegetables are a very important part of the macrobiotic diet, which has a long tradition of use in the natural treatment of disease.

# *Chapter Eight*

## RED IS THE NEW GREEN

While GMO's have infiltrated almost all non-organic corn, soy and wheat, and are now threatening the very existence of organic alfalfa, the sea plants are still wild, even when cultivated and have a primordial wisdom that these plants have developed over billions of years. And just as the form of the algae is dictated by its climate, depth, region and currents, so is its pigment. And just as purple cabbage contains "red chlorophyll" so do several species of R.M.A. or Red Marine Algae.  And just as the blue, green and red pigments have differences in color, these also have different phytochemistry and impact the body in a variety of beneficial ways. In this chapter we are going to examine some of the most promising discoveries from the oceans and waterways of this planet. While they have existed before man ever walked this earth, we are only now validating their importance in our development and survival. Because they have had to exist in a wet world where bacteria, viruses, mold and other parasites are common, they have developed defenses that may just connect humans to a level of wellness that eludes them. However to move forward into the future we must understand our past.

## "GREEN" FOODS THAT AREN'T

Here's some trivia about red cabbage: Although it's a deep purple color, it's really and truly a green food—because the purple pigments that give it its beautiful hue are photosynthetic pigments. Chlorophyll usually shows up as green, but it doesn't always show up that way. The flesh of a red cabbage is an excellent source of chlorophyll. The same goes for watermelon. The ruby-red, sweet flesh of that melon you cut open on a hot August afternoon is loaded with chlorophyll!

# RED MARINE ALGAE: THE ANTIVIRAL

Algae is at the bottom of the marine food chain, and is believed to be the earth's original plant. Fossil records show that algae has survived on this planet for around 3.5 billion years, virtually unchanged—a hardy, perfectly adapted and adaptable organism.

You've probably heard of other forms of algae used as food and medicine: blue-green algae, spirulina, and chlorella. You may not yet know about red marine algae, but it has been researched for over three decades due to the enormously promising antiviral properties of this plant.

Since the beginning of time, man has sought healing power from the plants of the earth. Only recently have modern scientists begun to scour the oceans in search of hidden secrets that may be valuable in industry or pharmacopeia. Tens of thousands of plants species have been collected and dissected as scientists, researchers and speculators all race to uncover the valuable natural resources that abound beneath the Sea. In the 1970's a major pharmacology company discovered a plant with unique qualities that they believed had the potential to be worth billions of dollars. A phytochemical unlike any they had seen before. A unique fusion of polysaccharides like those found in healing plants like aloe vera or noni, combined with sulfur compounds like those typically found in beets, broccoli and volcanic hotsprings. Together they formed a powerful sulfated polysaccharide, that in preliminary clinical studies showed an astounding anti-viral potential. While nearly all red colored seaweeds exhibit some anti-viral properties this is typically due to their content of carrageenans, a gummy substance typically found in edible red seaweed. However, not all carrageenan is created equal. You may say a red flag has been thrown up regarding Irish moss, a commonly used folk remedy which has now been implicated in inflammatory bowel responses triggered by its pathogenic foot print which, although non-toxic, over-stimulates our body's immune system thus leading to inflammation. Perhaps the research on red marine algae should be further clarified. At the very top of the feeding chain lie the gigartina and dumantacea varieties of algae. These rare, cold water species are the only edible varieties that contain the rare sulfated polysaccharides that we referred to in the pharmacological gold rush. It is the custom of the pharmacological industry to isolate and then chemically imitate the specific chemical sequences they discover within plants in order to patent them and to gain the exclusive rights to sell them, typically at whatever price the market will bear. And once they validated the amazing effect that these rare red marine algae species had on viruses (specifically the family of viruses referred to as Varicella-Zoster (chicken pox virus) which include herpes 1, herpes 2, shingles and mononucleosis) they naturally began the process of synthesizing them. Unfortunately, they were unable to do so. It seems that nature's ability to create this powerful phytochemistry was too much of a match after considering their alternatives, and they decided to abandon the project despite the millions of dollars spent on cultivation and research. Below are some examples of scientific research on these red algae that I believe validate their use as whole foods, either on the dinner plate or in supplement form.

It all started with intensive studies of marine organisms to locate potential sources of pharmacologically active agents. In a search for anti-herpetic substances, studies of California red marine algae proved to be particularly interesting. One study conducted by a Senior Research Fellow of the chemistry department at G.D. Searle & Co., Dr. Raphael Pappo, Ph.D., demonstrated the algae's beneficial effects on people with Herpes Simplex Virus I and II. Several years of study suggested to Dr. Pappo that the red marine algae assists the body's specific immune regulatory response and plays a key role in preventing the recurrence of the virus.

More recent research on extracts of red marine algae suggest that specific carbohydrates (sulfated polysaccharides) may inhibit both the DNA and RNA of viral infections and may operate both outside and within our infected cells. Work done in this area has shown sulfated polysaccharide compounds suppressed retroviral replication and inhibited viral reverse transcriptases. A study done by Neushul (1990) showed that nearly all of the 39 species of marine red algae, including the family Dumontiaceae, also contained and exhibited an inhibitory substance that suppressed retroviral replication and inhibited viral reverse transcriptases. Studies by Nakashima et al., (1987, 1988) support the hypothesis that a common immunomodulatory cell wall carbohydrate, like carrageenan, is a type of heparin receptor molecule, binding to a cell and triggering a specific cellular response sequence. Carrageenan may also be internalized into infected cells, thus inhibiting the virus. It also may inhibit fusion between infected cells suggesting that sulfated polysaccharides inhibit a step in viral replication subsequent to viral internalization but prior to the onset of late viral protein synthesis. In conclusion, the research indicates that the polysaccharides act as an immunomodulatory agent.

Because of the severity of the present AIDS epidemic and the debilitating effects of Herpes Simplex and Epstein-Barr, it is becoming more important than ever to re-examine the antiviral and immunomodulatory effects of red marine algae.

Additional research on red marine algae has shown promising results in the control and reduction of both the *Candida albicans* yeast (a fungus) and the *Herpes simplex* (virus simplexus), and it is becoming more important than ever to re-examine the antiviral and immunomodulatory effects that red marine algae may serve as a gateway to resist many other types of bacterial, fungal, and viral pathogens.

Just like the *demontacea*, the *Gigartina* genus of red marine algae is also rich in sulfated polysaccharides, or sulfur-containing complex sugars that have been found to improve the body's immune response.

These two rare red marine algae are rich in sulfated polysaccharides, which exhibit many biological properties such as antiviral and anticoagulant activities. In a general overview on red marine algae provided by researchers at the Naval Biosciences Laboratory, School of Public Health, University of California, Berkeley, it was noted that administration of red marine algae polysaccharides prevented death in 70 percent of mice receiving lethal amounts of murine pneumonia virus.

In a general overview on red marine algae from the Institute of Microbiology, Bulgarian Academy of Science, shows that an extract from red marine algae inhibited the reproduction of type 1 and type 2 herpes virus in cell cultures.

In 2004, Argentinean researchers published the results of a series of studies on red marine algae *carrageenans*—a type of polysaccharide, or complex carbohydrate, used to thicken foods like ice cream and soy milk. These researchers, at the University of Buenos Aires, repeatedly found antiviral actions of these carrageenans in mice infected with the herpes virus (HSV-II, the variant usually associated with genital herpes but that can also cause oral cold sores). Topical application of the carrageenan extract completely inhibited viral shedding—the route by which the virus is passed to others. Mice receiving topical red marine algae carrageenan had only 10 percent mortality following infection with HSV-II, while 9 of the 10 control mice died from complications of the virus. The other studies further supported the use of red marine algae as an antiviral agent against HSV strains I and II. Researchers can't use swabs made with calcium alginate in studies of viruses like herpes and chlamydia because of the alginate's toxicity to those viruses.

Other studies show that red marine algae inhibits replication of flu viruses and has general immune-stimulating properties, enhancing anti-body production. Its cell wall binds with toxic heavy metals in the body, which in excess can reduce the immune system's effectiveness at giving viruses the boot. Chlorella is also well known in the world of nutrition for this same effect. According to the research, using both algaes together is a good way to help reduce the impact of viruses on your life.

Red marine algae is a source of *alginates*, soluble fibers that bind tightly to radioactive substances like cadmium, sending them out of the body before they can do much damage. One Japanese study found that alginates could relieve symptoms of cadmium poisoning in people who had been poisoned by eating rice grown in cadmium-contaminated water. Alginates, like any other soluble fiber, can help reduce blood cholesterol levels and aid in the regulation of blood sugar levels.

Some research has suggested that alginates could be a useful therapy for gastroesophageal reflux disease (GERD). They form a gel-like physical barrier against the passage of stomach acids up into the esophagus. Alginates are used in some over-the-counter antacids.

## ASTAXANTHIN THE OTHER RED MARINE ALGAE

Astaxanthin is an equilateral hemocacus algae that survives in the warmest water on earth, yet can be found in cold waters as well. The intense sunlight, year round high temperatures, and gentle currents create one of the planet's true emocacus algato-chemicals. A deep red pigment that processes sunlight and protects the plant itself. If you have ever eaten shrimp, lobster or crab and noticed the bright red color or have seen the pink flesh of a wild salmon, you have seen astaxanthin. That pigment comes from a lifetime of eating algae. It helps them survive in cold waters and low sunlight. Farmed salmon by contrast have synthetic astaxanthin added to fool you. It has no nutritional value. The real astaxanthin however has a myriad of potential and proven benefits.

Astaxanthin is now being clinically proven to help in burning fat, reducing wrinkles, increasing energy, aiding in athletic recovery and performance, as a natural sunscreen antioxidant, and aiding in eye health and anti-aging.

## ASTAXANTHIN DEFENDS AGAINST REACTIVE OXYGEN SPECIES (ROS)

Oxygen present in our cells can form harmful radicals known as ROS or active oxygen when sufficient energy from UV rays is applied. ROS include singlet oxygen, superoxides and hydroxyl radicals (leading to peroxyl radicals) and they attempt to steal electrons from neighboring molecules such as DNA, phospholipids, enzymes and protein in order to stabilize. Fortunately, astaxanthin is able to quench singlet oxygen reactions and suppress lipid peroxidation much more effectively than other well-known antioxidants and thus control the presence of ROS. *In vitro* singlet oxygen quenching activity of Astaxanthin was found to be superior when compared to Catechin, Vitamin C, Alpha Lipoic Acid, Coenzyme Q10, Tocopherol, Lutein and Beta Carotene.

## WRINKLES

When most people see their own face in a magnifying mirror with a bright light, they can't believe how many "fine lines" and "micro wrinkles" they discover. Well, astaxanthin can make that experience a lot more pleasant.

Recent studies show:

Two human clinical trials established the use of astaxanthin to improve visible signs of premature aging and general skin health. The first, a double-blind placebo controlled study by Yamashita (2002), showed that astaxanthin in combination with tocotrienol, (a superior form of vitamin E), improved several aspects of overall skin condition. Eight female subjects with dry skin conditions (mean age 40 yrs.) received daily doses containing 2 mg astaxanthin and 40 mg natural tocotrienols. Several types of data were collected at 2 and 4 weeks and compared to the initial baseline readings. Measurable differences were observed starting just 2 weeks after supplementation. By the 4th week, the treated subjects with dry skin characteristics exhibited the following: increased moisture levels ($P<0.05$); consistent natural oils; reduction of fine wrinkles; and a reduction in pimples ($P<0.01$). Rice Bran Solubles are a great source of tocotrienols.

The second study by Yamashita (2006), female subjects with a variety of skin types (n=49, mean age 47 yrs.) were given either 4 mg (2 x 2 mg) astaxanthin or placebo in a single-blind, randomized, controlled study. After six weeks of consuming 4 mg astaxanthin per day, the results of a standard questionnaire showed that the treated group of women all felt that their skin condition had improved significantly (Figure 4).

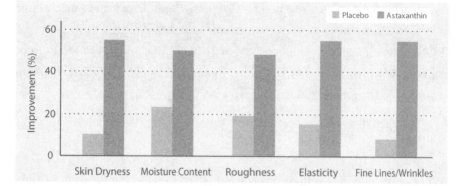

Figure 4. Subject response after 6 weeks astaxanthin supplementation.

Instrument analysis proved that the treated group had indeed achieved positive results in hydration ($P<0.05$) and elasticity ($P<0.05$). Furthermore, a dermatologist's inspection showed wrinkle reduction ($P<0.05$) and improved elasticity ($P<0.05$) in the treated group especially between weeks 3 and 6. The results were significant since skin regeneration usually takes between 4-5 weeks. The greatest improvement seen at week 6 supports the theory that astaxanthin protects and allows skin to regenerate

I love side effects, at least side effects like these. According to FDA studies, the average pharmaceutical drug has the negative side effect of weight gain. In fact an average of 15 additional pounds can be expected when taking 1 or more prescription drugs. People taking astaxanthin as part of clinical studies, however, for a variety of conditions reported they lost an average of 3 and a half pounds over 6 weeks. This is most likely due to the increased efficiency of energy production, and utilization at the cellular level.

Everyone needs more **energy** and our bodies know exactly how to give it to us, and it is not caffeine or other stimulants. It's glycogen, a simple combustible combination of glucose and oxygen. As long as our bodies produce glycogen we are fine. When it stops we suffer.

Do you worry about sun exposure? Have you ever tried to use sunscreen? Sticky sprays, creams, potions and lotions? Do you put it on your scalp where many melanomas develop? What about under your clothes? Do you know that sun light penetrates clothes and hair? What if I told you that there was an internal sunscreen that kept you ooey, gooey, sticky free! Well... astaxanthin.

## MECHANISM OF ACTION

Skin is composed of three layers: the epidermis, the dermis, and the subcutaneous fat. The dermis contains collagen, elastin, and other fibers that support the skin's structure. It is these elements that give skin its smooth and youthful appearance -- and these are the parts of the skin that are damaged by UV radiation (UVR).

# PROTECTING THE SKIN'S NATURAL ANTIOXIDANT NETWORK AND DNA

Oxygen radicals formed from UV radiation attack skin cells in a variety of ways. As demonstrated by O'Connor & O'Brien (1998), UVA light is capable of producing oxidative stress in living cells in-vitro. By monitoring catalase (CAT), superoxide dismutase (SOD) levels and thiobarbituric acid reactive substances (TBARS), astaxanthin is capable of reducing oxidative stress ($p < 0.01$, n=6) after UVA light irradiation at very low concentrations (5-10 nM). Astaxanthin has shown to be approximately 100-200 times more effective than other carotenoids, including lutein and beta-carotene ($1.0\ \mu M$).

Similar reports by Lyons *et al.*, (2002) demonstrate that UVA irradiated skin cells pretreated with astaxanthin ($10\ \mu M$) suffered significantly less DNA damage. Furthermore, astaxanthin protected the skin's endogenous antioxidants SOD and glutathione (GSH) from oxygen radical attack.

Weekend Warriors and professional athletes alike are rejoicing in this "discovery of recovery" due to its antioxidant and energy producing factors. But the real prize at the bottom of the box is the lack of soreness due to astaxanthin.

I always say, stress is stress. Whether the stress is caused by an extremely busy lifestyle, smoking, a poor diet, obesity, or and here's the kicker, physical exercise. All physical activity generates reactive oxygen species. The more physical activity you perform, or the greater stress that physical activity puts on your body, the more free radicals are created and the very exercise we are doing to make our muscles more attractive actually have a damaging effect and will ultimately effect performance and increase recovery times. As we know carotenoids protect both skin and muscle tissue, however they are fairly insignificant due to their low potency and long term actions. Astaxanthin, however, is a super carotenioid that acts quickly to increase endurance and muscle recovery time. Inside all of our cells are mitochondrial power producers which provide nearly all of our bodies' true energy, and by true energy I mean the property source of energy, burning glycogen and fatty acids inside of muscle tissue. During this combustion just like in an internal engine combustion engine, i.e. cars, trucks and motorcycles, there is a byproduct of exhaust. In the case of our cells, the exhaust is highly damaging, reactive oxygen. Reactive oxygen damages cells by triggering cell membrane peroxidation, and affect muscles long after the exercise has ceased. This is due to the inflammatory response caused by our immune system. The rapid monocytes response creates inflammation and additional muscle cell damage. This manifests during recovery in the form of tired, sore muscles. Modern athletes see astaxanthin as the antioxidant of choice. Which is not surprising since astaxanthin has demonstrated an ability to reduce muscle damage and increase endurance through improved lipid metabolism. In short, the reason why is because astaxanthin protects the outer muscle tissue from oxidative stress during physical activity. Meaning the endurance through improper from. And as an amazing and wonderful side effect, astaxanthin increases the metabolism of lipids to produce energy by transporting fat to the cells to be used as energy.

# ASTAXANTHIN BOOSTS ENDURANCE

In a randomized, double-blind, placebo controlled study on healthy men supplemented with 4 mg astaxanthin per day for up to 6 months at Karolinska Institute, Sweden, standardized exercise tests demonstrated that the average number of knee bends performed increased only in the astaxanthin treated group at 3 months, and by the 6 month significant improvements were observed. Furthermore, mice model studies by Ikeuchi *et al.*, (2006) showed that swimming endurance increased significantly ($p<0.01$) from one week of astaxanthin intake at 6 and 30 mg/kg body weight.

In another study, Aoi *et al.*, (2008) demonstrated that astaxanthin may modify muscle metabolism by its antioxidant property and result in improved muscle performance and weight loss benefits. After 4 weeks the mice running time to exhaustion had significantly improved by up to 20 % ($p<0.05$) with astaxanthin. In addition, Sawaki *et al.*, (2002) of Juntendo University, Japan, demonstrated by using 1200 meter track athletes, that a daily dose of 6 mg per day for 4 weeks resulted in their bodies accumulating lower levels of lactic acid. Ikeuchi *et al.*, (2006) also reported the same findings and furthermore, astaxanthin efficacy had a dose-dependent response.

In a double blind controlled placebo study, healthy women (n= 32; age-23-60) who ingested 12 mg of astaxanthin for 6 weeks significantly reduced their body fat (4%) when conducting routine walking exercise, compared to a placebo group. In addition, while control group increased their lactic acid by 31% compared to the astaxanthin group - only 13% ($p<0.05$). The same female participants who ceased oral administration of astaxanthin after the study were retested four weeks later and their body fat level rose again to the level observed at the start of study.

Aoi *et al.*, (2003) of Kyoto Prefecture University used mice models that may partially explain the efficacy of astaxanthin; they compared control, exercise placebo, and astaxanthin treated exercise groups after intense physical activity. 4-hydroxy-2-nonenal-modified-protein (4-HNE) stain analyses of the calf (gastrocnemius) muscles revealed significantly lower peroxidation damage.

The biochemical markers for oxidative damage and inflammation such as DNA ($p < 0.05$), creatine kinase ($p < 0.05$) and myeloperoxidase activity ($p < 0.05$) were significantly reduced in the astaxanthin treated exercise group. These effects indicate that astaxanthin has a role in helping protect muscle cell components and down modulating the inflammatory processes. Lee *et al.*, (2003) also explained that astaxanthin directly modulates inflammation caused by the release of the pro-inflammatory cytokines and mediators. *In vivo* and *in vitro* tests demonstrate that astaxanthin inhibits the IkB Kinase (IKK) dependent activation of the Nuclear Factor-kB (NF-kB) pathway, a key step in the production of pro-inflammatory cytokines and mediators.

Aoi *et al.*, (2008) also demonstrated increased lipid metabolism compared to carbohydrate as the main source of energy during strenuous activity. Furthermore, analysis of the mitochondrial lipid transport enzyme known as carnitine palmitoyltransferase I (CPT I) revealed increased fat localization and reduction of oxidative damage in the presence of astaxanthin. CPT I is important because it regulates fatty acyl-CoA entry into the mitochondria in the oxidation of fatty acids in muscle. Exercise-induced ROS may partly limit utilization of fatty acid via diminishing CPT I activity.

# Chapter Nine

## FOOD IS MORE THAN THE SUM OF ITS PARTS

*"When we eat in a healthy, harmonious way, our ability to attune and commune with the Divine is enhanced. To explore fully the relationship of nutrition to spiritual life, I had to evolve beyond the present materialistic mechanistic paradigm of nutrition to an expanded definition of nutrition that included subtle energetic principles. What is the purpose of nutrition? What is it we call nutrition? What is assimilated? What is that which is assimilating? What is the relationship between the nutrient assimilated and spiritual unfolding? What is the relationship between the nutrient that is taken in and the living system taking it in?"*

Gabriel Cousens, M.D., from *Spiritual Nutrition and the Rainbow Diet*

In the Essene Gospel, it says: "Then I put the awakened wheat into the soil of the angel of Earth, and the power of the Earthly Mother and all her angels entered into the wheat, and when the sun had risen four times the grains had become grass. I tell you truly, there is no greater miracle than this."

When I first discovered the phenomenon of green foods, I was fascinated by the huge disparity between the empirical evidence that green foods healed and the scientific evidence that attempted to explain how these various green plants regulate and normalize biological functions. The physiological, biochemical nuts and bolts of vitamins, minerals, and other substances isolated

159

from plants seemed to be only part of the picture of the healing power of green foods. There had to be a greater energy at work.

Doctors' accounts of miracle remissions, my own personal experience of healing myself from asthma (which no specialist or medicine had been able to help), and all the other stories I came across gave me the belief that there was more at work here than nutrients, calories, and fiber.

I began to study, read, and ask questions. As you know if you've read this far, my journey first led me to the Hippocrates Institute in Boston, where I had the privilege of learning from Ann Wigmore, the best-known American proponent of wheatgrass therapy. In her book, Ann took her explanations past vitamins and minerals and tried to explain how the proteins, enzymes, and chlorophyll in these alkaline, oxygenating green foods acted to help rejuvenate and normalize diseased bodies.

I also had the privilege of personally knowing and developing a working relationship with Dr. Bernard Jensen, the American father of iridology (the science of diagnosis through examination of the irises of the eyes) and avid researcher of chlorella. Eventually, for over six years I went to work for the Japanese pharmaceutical development company headed by Dr. Yoshihide Hagiwara. Dr. Hagiwara was the first to develop and study extensively the benefits of dried barley grass juice. Their work and the work of others mentioned in this book began to create in my mind a clearer picture of how green foods healed. Still, I wasn't satisfied, and I began to look for something more.

I knew instinctively that "life force"—*chi*—had as much to do with the benefits of green foods as any single vitamin or mineral. This led me to read two books that offered insight into the ways in which complex biological organisms benefit from consuming simple organisms like plants, enzymes, and bacteria.

The first book was *Biological Transmutations* by French scientist C. L. Kervran. This book explains how amazing living organisms are at creating balance, and how they actually manufacture and synthesize vital nutrients from seemingly unrelated substances—literally dismantling one kind of molecule to make another. The second book, *Spiritual Nutrition* by Gabriel Cousens, M.D., explores Subtle Organizing Energy Fields (SOEFs) and how they impact the quality of food, and, on a broader level, the link between spiritual and physical health.

Reading these books transformed my understanding of how food affects our bodies. I share this information with you in the hopes of further transforming your way of looking at the food you eat, and that this will turn you away from the foods that harm you and towards a greener way of life.

## BIOLOGICAL TRANSMUTATIONS

In plain English, biological transmutation is the transformation of one element (for example, magnesium) to another (for example, calcium) in the body—a transformation that mainstream science believes to be impossible. These theories emphasize that what foods do *in vivo* (in the body) is a different thing altogether from what foods do ex vivo (outside of the body). No analysis of a food done in a laboratory can give us a complete picture of what a food becomes when we ingest and digest it.

The spark of life adds a great deal to the nutritional quality of a food; most modern science lacks the tools with which to describe the way this spark alters the nutritive value of what we eat. In Professor Kervran's work, I found some of the only satisfying scientific explanations of this life force as it might apply to human nutrition—and to the healing power of green food.

A system of farming which sees plant foods as a conglomeration of isolated soil nutrients—that believes that healthy plants can grow from tired soil impregnated with artificial fertilizers—is doomed. *Real* food is shot through with energy, and the energy that is incorporated into green foods as they grow is a vital aspect of the nourishment with which they provide us. Humans (and their domesticated animal friends) are not adequately nourished on diets formulated by chemists with isolated doses of nutrients from fertilizers and with GMO tweaking that corrupts their genetic code. Eventually, such diets lead to deficiency diseases, because we need those extra energetic ingredients that only the natural cycle of plant life from rich soil can supply.

Any experienced gardener knows that skillful rotation of crops and sophisticated inter-cropping can do a great deal to keep up soil fertility and soil structure. Biological transmutations offer up the science of how this works. Even 45 years ago, when Professor Kervran wrote his landmark book, crop quality was already suffering as a result of chemically dependent monocultural farming that thinks it knows how to make food better than Mother Nature does.

Old-time farmers and organic farmers know that *the plant makes the soil*. It has been said that organic farming is really all about soil preparation. Nature knows how to maintain fertility in the soil—through the growth of self-colonizing plants, otherwise known as weeds. The weeds that grow in fields are rich in exactly the nutrients that soil requires.

For example, daisies are particularly calcium-rich. They tend to grow on lawns that lack calcium, and they add this mineral to the soil as they go through their life cycle. The most fascinating part of this is that *the daisies produce calcium when it is not available in the soil in which they grow*. They "create" calcium without having to draw it from the soil! This is at the root of Professor Kervran's research: that plants and animals can transmute certain nutrients into others that are required in their bodies or for the health of the soil in which they grow.

This is a revolutionary concept; for 200 years, science has believed that the energy required to transmute one element into another is far greater than what is available in biological systems like the human body or a plant. The theories describe a novel form of "cold fusion" that might be responsible for these transmutations—a very-low-energy nuclear reaction that happens at the cellular level.

One nineteenth-century researcher found that lawns stay healthy when provided with adequate calcium. When the calcium in the soil was exhausted, daises began to appear. He analyzed the ashes of these daises and found them to be rich in calcium. This led him to ask: Where does this calcium come from, if not from the soil? At that time, the question remained unanswered, but it piqued the interest of a lot of other investigators around the world.

French chemist Vauquelin showed that chicken only fed on grain excrete more calcium than they consume in the grain. The calcium appeared to have been created from some other mineral in the bodies of the chickens.

In 1822, an Englishman named Prout systematically studied variations in calcium in chicken eggs during incubation. Prout found that the chicks that hatched from those eggs contained four times more calcium than the eggs had contained; this provided evidence that the chicks were somehow transmuting another element into calcium. In Germany in 1849, Vogel germinated some seeds of watercress under highly controlled conditions; he found more sulfur in the sprouts than in the seeds from which they sprouted. And between 1856 and 1873, Lawes and Gilbert conducted experiments that showed that plants contained more magnesium than was available in the soil they grew from.

A crab can molt and make a new shell in only a day, in seawater that contains very little calcium. Analysis of the body of a molting crab has found that it contains only 3 percent of the calcium it would require to make a new shell. Hens deprived of calcium in their diets began to lay soft-shelled eggs; when fed purified mica, which is rich in potassium (not calcium), they scratched, rolled in, and pecked at it, and the following day their eggshells were hard again. The hens appeared to have transformed potassium into calcium.

Other researchers continue to demonstrate that there is something beyond basic chemistry that goes on energetically in the interaction of plants with soil—and the interaction of plants and animals who eat them.

## FOOD'S ENERGETIC FINGERPRINT: SOEFS

The concept of SOEFs, as described by physician Gabriel Cousens, M.D., is rooted in historical, cultural, spiritual, and scientific evidence extending back thousands of years.

For example, the Chinese science of acupuncture is based on meridians, energetic "pathways" that have been mapped all over the body. Along these meridians travels the subtle energy called *chi*. Chinese medicine is all about manipulation of chi along the meridians with acupuncture needles, moxibustion, and other therapies, creating or maintaining a state of energetic balance in the body. Foods strongly affect the balance of chi, and specific foods are prescribed to push that balance in a more healthful direction. In India, both the sciences of yoga and Ayurvedic medicine use the word *prana* to describe the subtle energy of bodies and the life force in other living fields. Foods have prana too, and can be used to affect the body's prana.

Further understanding that living systems are surrounded by subtle energy fields was greatly advanced by the discovery and use of Kirlian photography, a type of photography that shows us the form of SOEFs. An organic apple has a larger, more brilliant energy field than a conventionally grown apple. These are the subtle energy fields of these foods, and when we eat the food, we eat that energy, too. Living things have a larger, more brilliant energy field than things that are not alive.

To me, the most fascinating thing about SOEFs is that *they exist prior to the existence of the physical form*. They are not emanated from the physical form like the magnetic field line of a bar magnet. They are an organizing force—a cause, not an effect.

For now, even if you're skeptical, try to accept—even if just as a theoretical notion—that SOEFs exist and organize the form and function of both plant and human systems. This allows you to take an expanded view of food as having body, life force, and Subtle Organizing Energy Fields similar to those of the human body. It is the dynamic interaction of these human and plant SOEFs that is important in understanding the new paradigm of "wholistic" nutrition.

SOEFs are only one part of the puzzle. Dr. Cousens' theories of spiritual nutrition aim to help us understand the interactions of nutrition, longevity, consciousness, and energy centers in the body (chakras). His work focuses on the link between the food we eat and our spiritual health.

# SPIRITUAL NUTRITION: EAT YOUR ENERGY!

Based on the work of such scientific luminaries as Albert Einstein and Nikolai Tesla, scientists are developing theories that matter is created through the condensation of subtle energetic vibrations that are happening everywhere, all the time. SOEFs are an attempt to describe how this precipitation from subtle energy to material form takes place, and how it is ordered. The study of how this energy affects our health is thousands of years old.

All living organisms are infused with a life force or energy; this force or energy can be influenced by other energetic vibrations. According to the theories that are the basis of SOEFs, these vibrations are a sort of "template" on which the material world is built.

This unseen energy is as essential to life as the air we breathe. In our materialistic world, this notion of energy is sometimes difficult to grasp and accept. It's regarded with suspicion by mainstream thought and medicine. But as mainstream thought and medicine become less and less appealing— as we learn more about their risks and the benefits of natural therapies— more and more people are becoming aware of subtle currents of energy in the foods they consume, in their bodies, and in the world they inhabit. This rising consciousness is one of the driving factors behind the current strong movement toward alternative medicine.

Over the centuries, healers and physicians have discovered and used many different forms of energy healing using light, color, and sound. The energies of plants, flowers, minerals, and even animals are used to positively influence the energetics of the human body. Ancient Greek mathematician Pythagoras once referred to a rock as an "orchestra of energy." Since—and, probably, before—that time, artists, mystics, and scientists have sought to describe the energetic qualities of objects both animate and inanimate. Manifestations of that energy have been the subject of works of art throughout history; Native American totem sculptures, aboriginal rock paintings, and ancient Indian sculptures all represent it with an *aura*, an energy field that surrounds the physical body.

# ELECTROMAGNETIC FORCE FIELDS: NOT JUST FOR SCI-FI TV

In the mid-1940s, Dr. Harold Saxton Burr, an American researcher and anatomy professor at Yale University Medical School, shattered conventional belief with his development of the *electrodynamic theory of life*. This theory suggested that all physical forms are held together and managed by electromagnetic fields of energy. Dr. Burr called these electromagnetic fields *life-fields*, or L-fields for short. He stated that these L-fields, which could be measured quite easily with standard voltmeters, are the basic blueprint of life on earth; and, he believed that medicine should be able to use measurements of the L-fields to diagnose illness before symptoms develop.

It sounds like bad sci-fi, something out of *Star Trek* or *Lost in Space*, but Dr. Burr was no TV writer, and definitely not a member of any fringe element; he was a Professor Emeritus at Yale who published 93 academic papers in his 43 years at that esteemed institution. His work on L-fields is highly respected even today, and helps to explain why flower essences and other vibrational therapies work so well. Many modern scientists, including Candace Pert, Ph.D. (who wrote about her life's work on mind-body medicine in her best-selling book *Molecules of Emotion*), Dr. Richard Gerber, Robert D. Becker, M.D., and Ervin Laszlo, continue to study the energetic patterns that occur within the body and how they are influenced by our thoughts and states of illness or well-being, and vice-versa.

According to Dr. Burr, the L-field is highly sensitive. It responds to energy impulses within the environment. Dr. Burr describes electrodynamic fields in his classic book, *Blueprint for Immortality* (C.W. Daniel Company, Ltd., 2004), as "invisible and intangible," and uses the analogy of the typical high-school science project involving magnets, a card, and some iron filings. When the filings are scattered over the card while the magnet is underneath, they arrange themselves in the pattern of that magnet's lines of force. If you remove the filings and put new filings on the card, they arrange themselves in exactly the same way.

Burr posits that the same thing happens in the human body. Our molecules and cells are, he states, "constantly being torn apart and rebuilt with fresh material from the food we eat. But, thanks to the controlling L-fields, the new molecules and cells are rebuilt as before and arrange themselves in the same pattern as the old ones." Until voltammetry and other modern instruments revealed the existence of L-fields, science could not explain how our bodies knew how to continually re-form new tissues in exactly the right configurations despite the relentless turnover of material in the body. Burr describes the L-fields as matrices or molds that "preserve...the 'shape' or arrangement of any material poured into it, however often the material may be changed." He uses the analogy of a jelly mold, into which you can pour jelly to form into a shape as it sets. If there is something wrong with the mold—a dent or bulge, for example—the resulting mold has a dent or a bulge, too. Flaws in the energetic field create flaws in the body that forms within it. Some of the experiments performed or described by Burr found that cancerous growths in the ovary could be revealed through L-field measurements before any other signs or symptoms appeared.

In *Blueprint for Immortality*, Burr writes about the research of Dr. Louis Langman of New York University and Bellevue Hospital Gynecological Service. They "examined over 1,000 patients using electro-metric measurements of the L-field," then "examined patients who were on the wards of the hospital and were subject to a variety of syndromes. They included fibromas, as well as the usual run of pathological events in the generative tract of these women. In those that showed a marked change in the voltage gradient between the cervix and the ventral abdominal wall, careful watch was kept through subsequent laparotomy...there were a hundred and two cases where there was a significant shift in the voltage gradient, suggesting malignancy. Surgical confirmation was found in ninety-five of the one hundred and two cases. The actual position of the malignancy varied all the way from the fundus, to the tubes and to the ovarian tissue itself. We had an astonishingly high percentage of successful identification of malignancy in the generative tract, confirmed by biopsy."

Fascinating stuff. It suggests that energy fields are not only full of potential for the balancing of human physiology and prevention of disease, but also for very, very early diagnosis of some of the most feared conditions that afflict modern humans.

You're getting just a taste of the science that has been done to give us insight into how life force or living energy contributes to a plant's nutritional value. Another researcher, Dr. Fritz-Albert Popp from Germany, actually developed a method of measuring this life force that he calls *biophotonic emission testing*, that takes Kirlian photography to the next level.

Dr. Fritz-Albert Popp is a well-known biophysicist and professor at Kaiserslautern University in Germany. His research began with the confirmation of the existence of *biophotons*, which are electromagnetic waves emitted by living organisms. Biophotons cannot be seen by the naked eye, but they can be measured by sensitive modern equipment. Dr. Popp found that this phenomenon is common to all forms of cells, and that if they are in a healthy condition, they emit more than they do when in an unhealthy condition.

Biophotonic measuring techniques offer an extremely sensitive, noninvasive, holistic, powerful tool for investigating and understanding the quality of food and of the environment.

## MEDICINAL MARIJUANA: A REPORT

One of the most compelling and unjust issues that I have been trying to get attention for over the past few years for mental and physical issues in the **health industry**, is the legalization of medicinal marijuana. Whether you agree or disagree or just aren't sure, it is time to talk, review, debate and explore. When and how did it all begin? What are the options being presented to the people most likely to benefit from this alternative form of medicine? What could be the repercussions? These will be discussed in the next few pages and hopefully will provide you with a deeper insight on this often delicate and contentious subject.

As a child growing up in the inner-city, it was very obvious that marijuana was a vital part of the local "economy". While very few opportunities existed for employment and upward mobility it seemed as though that a few enterprising and entrepreneurial individuals had created an industry of their own. They were the ones with the nice clothes, big cars, and fat wallets. And

I noticed that many young men from my neighborhood ended up in jail for participating in this enterprise. I saw it as a great disparity in the application of the law when, what was to me a substance quite similar to alcohol in that it caused intoxication and like cigarettes, was consumed through combustion. Yet it was illegal, and those who ingested, distributed, imported or grew the substance were criminals in the eyes of the law, their families, and future employers. Hundreds of millions, in fact billions of dollars were being spent to prevent the use of marijuana and to jail the participants in that industry. Meanwhile, roads went unfixed, people went hungry, and our government was going bankrupt trying to support the industry of keeping people behind bars. Over 50% of the prisoners in many cities, counties and states are there for a victimless crime, for using a substance that may in fact turn out to be not only safe and harmless, but in fact one of the greatest gifts of nature. One that has the ability to fight stress, anxiety, seizures, traumatic brain injuries and maybe even cancer! The following is an unbiased reporting of the history of hemp, cannabis and marijuana. Keep your mind open, it is a brave new world.

## HEMP BY ANY OTHER NAME IS STILL... CANNABIS

Strictly speaking, **Cannabis** is a genus of flowering plants that includes three different species, *Cannabis sativa*, *indicia* and *ruderalis*. **Hemp**, on the other hand, is the commonly used term for the high-growing varieties of this plant family, which are mainly cultivated for its fibrous material and edible parts (seeds and oils), and contains almost none of the properties associated with pot, weed or marijuana.

Cannabis is also used for medicinal purposes and as a recreational drug. It is the preparation of the cannabis plant intended for use as a psychoactive drug and as a medicine that is labeled as **marijuana**.

The Cannabis plant hosts a complex variety of chemical compounds, some of which are unique to the species. For example, out of the 483 compounds identified, more than 60 cannabinoids have been classified as singular to the plant family. The term "**cannabinoids**" represents a group of $C_{21}$ terpenophenolic compounds that, up to now, has not been found anywhere else but in this flowering plant family.

It is from these cannabinoids that the "high" one experiences from consuming marijuana comes from. The two cannabinoids that are produced in the greatest abundance are cannabidiol (CBD) and $\Delta^9$-tetrahydrocannabinol (THC), but only the latter is psychoactive. Curiously, CBD has recently been found to block the effect of THC in the nervous system. The varying amounts of the two cannabinoids in the different species of the plant may produce different effects in humans. Cannabis *sativa* has a higher level of THC compared to CBD, while Cannabis *indica* has a higher level of CBD compared to THC. Cannabis varieties that have a relatively high CBD to THC ratios are less likely to induce anxiety and vice versa. Popularly, *sativa* is well known for the cerebral "high" that it produces while *indica* is known for its sedative effects.

## CAN CANNABIS CURE CANCER?

With the extremely restrictive laws surrounding the distribution of marijuana for research and medical use, licensed growers are currently developing more CBD-rich strains. In November 2012, Tikun Olam, an Israeli medical cannabis facility, formally announced a new strain of the plant which only has cannabidiol as an active ingredient, and virtually no THC, allowing the administration of the medicinal benefits of the plant without the euphoria. This new strain has been announced to be a viable treatment for rheumatoid arthritis, colitis, liver inflammation, PTSD, fibromyalgia, heart disease, cancer and diabetes. As of February 2014, a patent application for the new hybrid named "avidekel" has been filed.

## THE HISTORICAL "HIGH" OF MARIJUANA. WHILE THE ROCKY MOUNTAINS ARE THE MODERN PLAY ON GETTING "HIGH"

Cannabis is believed to have originated in the mountainous regions northwest of the Himalayas and is accepted as endemic to Central and South

Asia but has spread widely. Cannabis *sativa* in particular appears naturally in many tropical and humid parts of the world. Its use as a medicine has both been a subject of local folklore and documented by archeological finds in prehistoric societies throughout the world.

As far back as 2900 BC, marijuana has been referenced as popular medicine in China along with the likes of ginseng and ephedra. The Chinese Emperor, Fu Hsi, was quoted to have remarked that cannabis possessed both yin and yang, the two governing forces of life as taught by their traditional philosophies. By 200 BC, cannabis combined with resin and wine was popularly used as an anesthetic during surgical procedures.

It is also believed that the anointing oil most frequently referred to in the Old Testament is largely made up of *kaneh-bosem* which, in the original Hebrew version of the recipe in Exodus, is recognized to be cannabis by many etymologists, linguists, and other researchers. This extends to the anointing oil that Jesus used in the New Testament for his followers.

Ancient prescriptions unearthed in Egypt included cannabis used for treatment of glaucoma, inflammation, and cooling the uterus, as well as in the administration of enemas.

By 1000 BC, the use of cannabis as a medicine for a wide variety of ailments had spread to India. People believed it could boost mental abilities and judgment, promote longevity, lower fevers, cure insomnia, leprosy, and dysentery, among others. A cannabis-milk infusion called *bhang* became popular as an anesthetic and anti-phlegmatic. By 600 BC, the uses of cannabis were laid out in the Ayurvedic treatise of Sushruta Samhita.

In the ancient western civilization, the earliest written records of cannabis usage is by the Greek historian, Herodotus, and was a part of his famous book, Histories (circa 400 BC). He referred to the Scythians' tradition of taking cannabis steam baths that elicited such euphoric reactions from those who smelled the marijuana-infused vapors. By 200 BC, the Greeks were using marijuana as a remedy for earache, edema, and inflammation. The use of medicinal marijuana later on spread to the Romans by way of the Greek physician, Pedanius Dioscorides, who served as an army doctor in Rome. In his book *De Materia Medicae*, he referred to "that plant which was used in the making of rope" as capable of producing a juice that could suppress sexual longing. This was later on supported by Pliny the Elder in his writings, further adding gout, cramped joints, and similar muscular pains as ailments cured by the roots of the cannabis plant boiled in water.

The use of marijuana medicinally continued its advance across both eastern and western civilizations during the Middle Ages, when it was considered one of the most important contents of any herbalist's medicine cabinet. Nausea, parasitic infections, hemorrhage, diarrhea, dysentery, and poor appetite were added to the long list of ailments supposedly cured by marijuana. Chinese folk medicine, in particular, favored the medicinal plant greatly.

## OUR FIRST PRESIDENT GREW POT?

The marijuana plant, then commonly known as hemp, crossed the Atlantic to North America in 1611 when it was brought over by the Jamestown settlers as an important export item to be cultivated in the new colonies for the fiber that it produced. Later on, its medicinal properties regained its original popularity that even famous statesmen such as George Washington and Thomas Jefferson grew them on their properties.

Back in Europe, Napoleon brought back marijuana to France from his invasion of Egypt and became more widely accepted as a pain reliever in western medicine. By 1840, cannabis was reintroduced into British medicine by Dr. W. O'Shaughnessy from his military servitude in India. It was widely used to treat various ailments such as muscle spasms, menstrual cramps, rheumatism, and the convulsions of tetanus, rabies, and epilepsy. It was also used to promote uterine contractions during childbirth and as a sedative. Marijuana was administered orally in the form of a tincture and its extracts were also incorporated in many different medicines at that time.

## UP UNTIL 80 YEARS AGO MARIJUANA WAS MEDICINE

The 19th Century saw marijuana emerge as a mainstream medicine in the West. By 1850, it was officially added to the United States Pharmacopeia and patented marijuana tinctures were sold as popular cures for various afflictions such as neuralgia, tetanus, typhus, cholera, rabies, dysentery, alcoholism, opiate addiction, anthrax, leprosy, incontinence, gout, convulsive disorders, tonsillitis, insanity, excessive menstrual bleeding, and uterine bleeding.

The popularity of marijuana at that time didn't mean that it didn't have any detractors. In fact, it was due to the concern over the plant being an intoxicant that led to the establishment of the Indian Hemp Commission of 1893-1894 to examine the use of cannabis in India. Ironically, this led to further research into more medicinal properties of the controversial plant and ultimately establishing its value in the Indian subcontinent where it is still widely being used in rural areas as a medicine.

## THE BEGINNINGS OF CONTROVERSY

Strangely enough, the start of the regulation of marijuana in the United States was not sparked by similar concerns over its psychoactive properties, but due to other prevailing social and political issues at that time that were completely unrelated. Take into example the passing of the Wiley Act in 1906 by then-President Roosevelt to require the labeling of medicine being sold, including cannabis. This law was drafted with more concern over the regulation of product labeling than pre-market approval.

Even in the Prohibition Era of the 1910's, marijuana was not one of the primary concerns of the legislature as it tackled moral issues such as liquor, prostitution, racetrack gambling and prizefighting. It was only as part of regulatory initiatives to discourage future use why some states, Massachusetts being the first, had begun to ban cannabis beginning from 1911 through 1917.

## TAXES, TAXES, TAXES

In January 1915, the future model for future drug regulation legislation came about when President Woodrow Wilson passed the Harrison Act, which required all physicians who prescribed opium or any of its derivatives to put a serial number, which could be obtained from the Internal Revenue Department, on each prescription. This was aimed to allow for the imposition of special taxes upon persons who sell, distribute or give away opium or coca leaves. The act also controlled the opium trade so that it would only allow the sale of the plant and its extracts for medicinal purposes. Although the law did not apply to marijuana, this is considered to have been the basis of all future drug regulatory actions.

The growing pressure on the trade and use of marijuana shifted to the international scene on February 19, 1925, when the League of Nations signed a multilateral treaty restricting cannabis use to scientific and medical only. Furthermore, cannabis was added to the United Kingdom's list of prohibited drugs under its Dangerous Drugs Act in 1928.

Despite the growing international concern over the use of cannabis as a psychoactive drug, the United States continued to tolerate the regulated use of the plant in medicinal preparations, even going as far as becoming a self-sufficient producer of homegrown cannabis through pharmaceutical farms east of the Mississippi. Pharmaceutical companies like Parke-Davis and Eli Lily were able to meet the growing demand for cannabis-based medicine with their standardized extracts of the plant for use as an analgesic, an antispasmodic, and a sedative.

It was only in 1930 at the appointment of Harry J. Anslinger as Commissioner of the Federal Bureau of Narcotics that the status of cannabis as an established medicinal plant suffered an inexorable blow. Fueled by sensationalized crime reports, bloated statistics and tinges of xenophobia, Anslinger launched an all-out-war against marijuana in his fourth year as commissioner. His campaign rested on two fantastical assertions: that the drug caused insanity; and that it pushed people toward horrendous acts of criminality.

It has been alleged that the attack on cannabis in the 1930's had hidden agendas by its main proponents. Anslinger received a fairly hefty amount of support and mass media coverage from newspaper mogul, William Randolph Hearst. Hearst had reportedly large investments in the lumber and paper industries, thus taking out hemp as an industrial competitor would not be above his motivation for dipping into the smear campaign against marijuana. Many of the most outlandish stories linking violent acts to cannabis consumption appeared in his newspapers.

Aside from the tremendous bad press that cannabis was receiving at that time, the development of new drugs such as aspirin, morphine, and other highly addictive opium-derived medication hastened the decline for the demand of medicinal marijuana. This was compounded by the Marihuana Tax Act of 1937 which, like the Harrison Act, required medical professionals who prescribed or dispensed marijuana to register with federal authorities and pay an annual tax or license fee. Prescriptions of marijuana naturally declined with the extra work and fees faced by medical practitioners when cheaper, less worrisome alternatives were available.

Despite this, cannabis did not have a shortage in support from people who had first-hand information about its pharmacological value. The American Medical Association was a staunch opponent of the Marihuana Tax Act, arguing during the hearings prior to the law's passing, that restricting the use of cannabis by a prohibitive tax would prevent future investigation of more substantial medical uses of cannabis. New York City Mayor, Fiorello LaGuardia, also debunked the exaggerated dangers of marijuana by way of the "LaGuardia Report", an investigative report about marijuana, which he requested from the New York Academy of Medicine in 1938.

Nevertheless, the unrelenting anti-marijuana sentiment raised by the likes of Anslinger and Hearst paved the way for the law to be enacted by Congress. By 1942 marijuana was removed from the US Pharmacopeia, finally relegating the once-valued plant to the ranks of illicit substances. By 1970 it was placed in Schedule I under the Controlled Substances Act categorizing marijuana as "having a high potential for abuse, no currently accepted medical use in treatment in the United States, and a lack of accepted safety for use of the drug or other substance under medical supervision."

## THE FIGHT FOR LEGALIZATION

The classifying of cannabis as a Schedule I substance under the CSA did not by any means end the fight for people who believed in its beneficence.

Independent bodies such as the American College of Physicians and the American Medical Association have been clamoring for the US government to reconsider its classification of marijuana as a Schedule I substance under the rationale that further research on the plant as a whole is required to come to an objective conclusion about the merits and evils of cannabis.

Although the status of marijuana on the federal government level has stayed relatively the same since the 1970's, largely due to the unyielding stance of DEA & NIDA, its situation at the state level has since greatly improved.

In 1996, California passed an initiative to allow medical cannabis. By June 2014, New York became the 23rd state to legalize medical marijuana (excluding DC). Though each state's marijuana regulations vary in terms of method of usage, distribution, possession, etc., it still served as a unifying force in the marijuana movement as it renewed debates on the legality of the federal government's continuing prohibition and its relevance to newer findings on the plant's medicinal value. A 2010 ABC News poll showed that 81 percent of Americans believed that medical cannabis should be legal in the United States.

Congress passed a measure on May 29, 2014, that would deny the Drug Enforcement Agency to spend federal money interfering with state approved medical marijuana businesses. A month later, Senators Rand Paul and Cory Booker offered similar amendments to prevent the Department of Justice and the DEA from using their government funding to undermine states that have legalized marijuana. This came after a slew of complaints from Massachusetts doctors who claim to have been threatened with loss of license by the DEA if they continue prescribing marijuana.

As long as the federal and state level maintain their disparity over medical marijuana legalization, this scenario will continuously play itself out across the nation, with patients relying on cannabis getting caught in the middle.

## LAB WORKS

Ever since cannabis has been placed in Schedule I, there has almost been no clinical research done in the United States regarding the therapeutic benefits of the plant. The only entity legally authorized to approve contracts to grow cannabis and distribute them for research purposes was the National Institute on Drug Abuse. The government agency has been under fire for the longest time from independent research groups for an alleged refusal to supply the plant to researchers who had already obtained all other necessary federal permits.

Presently, researchers are making do with existing studies on the therapeutic benefits of marijuana conducted in other countries with more lenient regulations on marijuana supply, as well as studying patients who have already been certified for medical use of cannabis, or otherwise use synthetic cannabinoids such as JWH-018 to replicate the effects. The latter proved to be a failure as the chemical had been reported to be five times more potent than natural THC found in the cannabis plant, thus results obtained from using the synthetic option are not comparable to that of the natural substance. This also led to the substance infiltrating the illicit drug market, thereby worsening the already-besmirched image of the natural marijuana.

The available knowledge on the medical uses of cannabis and cannabinoids is, at best, marked by differences due to the stunted progress of its research. For the treatment of nausea and vomiting associated with cancer chemotherapy, chronic (especially neuropathic) pain, spasticity in multiple sclerosis and spinal cord injury, and anorexia and cachexia in HIV/AIDS, strong evidence of the plant's medical benefits have been made available through existing studies. However, marijuana's efficacy for other indications such as epilepsy, pruritus and depression require further investigation.

Due to limited means of systematic research, much of the benefits of medical marijuana have been found through clinical research inspired by positive feedback from patients using crude cannabis products. Such is the case for the recognition of marijuana's anti-emetic, appetite-enhancing, relaxing and analgesic effects, and therapeutic use in Tourette's syndrome. This kind of study usually leads to the incidental observation of more therapeutically useful effects. Similarly, this was how marijuana has been found to decrease the disturbed behavior among patients with Alzheimer's disease when they were originally being observed for the appetite-stimulating effects of THC. This was also the method on how THC was discovered to alleviate intraocular pressure for glaucoma patients back in the 1970's. Due to this trend, the primary source of knowledge for marijuana's medicinal benefits has turned towards the empirical method of patient/user surveys though not as desirable as controlled clinical trials.

Researchers are being hopeful though, as the current efforts to decriminalize marijuana rage on, new studies bring to light newer and more substantial evidence in favor of medical marijuana. One such development is the research done at the Los Angeles Biomedical Research Institute on patients with traumatic brain injuries.

The findings, released in October 2014, suggest that THC may help protect the brain in cases of traumatic brain injury. The study included 446 patients who suffered traumatic brain injuries and underwent a urine test for the presence of THC in their system. The researchers found 82 of the patients had THC in their system. Of those, only 2.4% died. Of the remaining patients who didn't have THC in their system, 11.5% died. The study was one of the first in a clinical setting to specifically associate THC use as an independent predictor of survival after a traumatic brain injury.

## DON'T GET HIGH, GET JUICED!

Another recent development is the catching on of marijuana to a popular nutritional trend nowadays... juicing. There are several proponents of this technique of imbibing the benefits of marijuana, such as Dr. Donald

Abrams, chief of Hematology and Oncology at the San Francisco General Hospital, and Dr. William Courtney, Vice President of the Association Luxembourgeoise des Methodes Preventives, an ambulatory care facility in Luxembourg, utilizing dietary unheated cannabis. They believe that the absence of heat in the preparation of medicinal marijuana allows the consumer to receive the most nutritional benefits of the plant without the "high" that is usually associated with smoking or vaporizing it. Dr. Courtney believes that cannabis can assist in the function of the human immune system, provide anti-inflammatory benefits, and improve bone metabolism and neural function. Cannabis could also inhibit cancer cell growth, according to the doctor.

In the international scene, a 2014 research done by specialists at St. George's University in London has shown evidence that THC and CBD combined with irradiation therapy in lab mice with brain tumors had drastically slowed down the growth of the malignancies.

Cannabinoids have long been recognized as effective in counteracting the side effects of antineoplastic therapy, including chemotherapy, but the effect of the cannabis plant elements on actual tumors is something new and the research is now gearing towards actual human clinical trials. This is a very important breakthrough as brain cancer is particularly difficult to treat and claims the lives of about 5,200 people each year.

Similarly, another study published in September 2014 has added evidence to the benefits of marijuana in the treatment of Alzheimer's disease.

As with cancer, marijuana had long been recognized to help Alzheimer's disease patients by increasing their appetite. But with this new study cannabinoids take on a greater role in the treatment of the sixth leading cause of death in the US.

Researchers at the University of South Florida and Thomas Jefferson University were able to observe that THC was effective at lowering Amyloid-$\beta(A\beta)$ levels in treated Alzheimer's research cells. $A\beta$ is a type of protein linked to Alzheimer's symptoms. As THC has been established as a natural and relatively safe amyloid inhibitor, the research group is hopeful that this new finding will be instrumental in developing an effective treatment in the future.

## IN CONCLUSION

Marijuana has come a long way from being just "that plant which was used in the making of rope". After spending centuries being celebrated as a potent cure for a majority of mankind's ailments, it only took a few years of bad press and rash judgment for the controversial plant to go from indispensable to illicit.

Despite the torrent of new findings on the benefits of cannabis, there is still a lot of room for further study as many areas in the use of the plant are still gray. In the ongoing campaign to make medical marijuana legally available to patients who will benefit from its properties, every ounce of solid, scientifically-backed evidence is important. The stereotype and old wives' tales built around the use of marijuana has all but demolished its image, if not for the legacy of cures it has built for itself prior to its period of prohibition. As Dr. Adams quoted, *"If cannabis were discovered in the Amazon rainforest today, people would be clambering to make as much use as they could of all of the potential benefits of the plant. Unfortunately, it carries with it a long history of being a persecuted plant."*

## SCARED STRAIGHT

In the attempt to keep youth from experimenting with drugs, particularly marijuana, the following was seen by millions of teenagers in high schools across America.

The Scene: Teenager is seen smoking pot with his friends and then experiences a "bad trip". Believing he can fly he climbs to the top of a high building and jumps to his death... In reality there is almost no link to hallucinations, violent behavior or suicidal thoughts associated with cannabis use. But this image will be indelibly etched in our minds.

# PURE FOOD CRISIS

I always say the quality of the food we eat, will equal the quality of the life we live. Naturopathy, a 2500 year old tradition, is based upon the philosophy that the human body is capable of achieving perfect health or homeostasis, if it is fed and cared for properly. I firmly believe that human beings have the ability and the responsibility to maximize the potential of their existence, and that they can only do so if they take extreme care in the selection, preparation and consumption of their sustenance, AKA the food which keeps them alive. It is for that reason that I feel compelled to rally the troops, to sound the alarm, to warn all of you about this impending danger, this threat to our very existence. The threat to the very food that nourishes us. The threat that I call the Pure Food Crisis. As I have stated before, the Pure Food Crisis had its roots in both the creation of the Chicago Board of Trade, as well as the creation of commercial canning of food. The Chicago Board of Trade, or CBOT, was established in the late 1800's and was designed to distribute food across cities, states, and the entire country, and required the mass production of standardized food. Inevitably the stabilizers, preservatives and chemicals required to create this mass uniformity were created in order to sustain this distribution model. When food became a commodity to be traded like gold and silver, the emphasis on its ability to sustain life diminished and the emphasis on its ability to sustain profitability expanded. Ultimately, the interest of corporations began to outweigh the interest of consumers and a silent conspiracy between the seed companies and the pesticide companies ultimately resulted in experimentation that in many people's minds have crossed the boundaries of safety and sanity.

# SAY NO TO GMO'S

I want to make a statement about GMO's, just so that everyone understands. Most of the world has rejected GMO's and has chosen to act cautiously. Only a few nations (that are influenced by the companies that have the most to gain) have chosen to allow their populations to be exposed to this potential danger. Unfortunately, the United States is one of them. There have been NO significant safety studies required before these sophisticated and potentially dangerous bio-organisms were unleashed, not only into the delicate ecosystem, but more frighteningly into the more delicate ecosystem we call the human body. We have learned through drug trials that even when something appears safe in initial limited exposures, when the exposure grows to the general population, much more is revealed; even though none of the aforementioned human studies were ever performed, the ultimate epidemiological study is being played out in our vulnerable and unsuspecting human population. In an incredible continuation of the total disregard for consumer safety, the fact that GMO's are in your foods is being hidden from you through legislation that protects the mega corporations from having to label these foods as containing GMO's, JUST as we have done with trans fats, salt, gluten, peanuts, and other ingredients where consumer safety is of concern.

To be 100% clear, potentially dangerous GMO's are in your food right now and you don't even know it. One of the major battle grounds in the fight to properly regulate and label genetically modified foods is the Island State of Hawaii. Grass roots movements on both Maui and Kauai have seen motivated voters demand that the agribusinesses play fair and not gamble with the future health of their children, or their homeland. New voter approved legislation would require full disclosure when a crop or field is being used to produce GMO's, as well as safety zones or buffers that keep dangerous chemicals away from schools, houses, hospitals and businesses where vulnerable populations can be exposed to them. Despite these democratically mandated safety regulations, the billion dollar corporations have unleashed an army of lawyers and a barrage of misinformation attempting to divide the population by promising jobs and prosperity without revealing the long term dangers to those who both work with and consume these manmade "Frankenfoods".

Five decades ago, a call to action resonated across the nation to rouse citizens against the long-lasting hazards of pesticides, DDT in particular, not only to the environment but especially to people's health. Renowned nature author and former marine biologist Rachel Carson wrote the book *Silent Spring* and published it in 1962 (the year I was born coincidentally) to awaken the nation about pesticides, ultimately leading to DDT being banned in the US.

A powerful call to action like this is once more in order at this point in time to bring us together in a collective movement against so-called people of science. Those who have sold their principles to GMO giants like Monsanto to propagate tampered "proof" that GMO's in our food are safe and the only solution to feeding a ballooning population. It can be recalled that even in the time of Carson, Monsanto was also the main proponent of a subtle black propaganda against the author in an attempt to counteract *Silent Spring's* immense impact to Americans. Fortunately, there was still a proliferation of principled scientists at that time who were not afraid of corporate blackballing and rose to the author's defense, effectively vindicating her and further validating the potency of her work. Unfortunately, this is no longer the case as their counterparts nowadays are the people behind the laboratory-spun lies made in the name of corporate greed that fuels the GMO debacle.

Additionally, GMO's are threatening the very existence of organic agriculture. All organic farmers rely upon alfalfa as either a source nitrogen building green manure or as an effective cover crop. Unfortunately, GMO alfalfa has the ability to quickly cross pollinate and compromise the organic status of alfalfa on the entire continent, driving the price of organic vegetables, meats and fruits to unprecedented levels due to a lack of inexpensive nitrogen based fertilizer, once alfalfa can no longer be used. The ability of legumes, which are perennials, to create nitrogen fixation and thus naturally fertilize organic crops is vital to every organic farmer's ability to survive.

## RHIBOZIUM, SECRETS OF THE SOIL

Nitrogen... every plant needs it to grow. To grow a lot of plants you need a lot of nitrogen. But where will it come from? Well, in modern agriculture it usually comes from chemical fertilizers, and/or manure which comes from commercial cattle or other livestock. In organic agriculture, it typically comes from an amazing synergistic relationship between a parasitic soil organism and the alfalfa plant, which not only provides nitrogen to the organism and its host, but also is capable of releasing excess nitrogen in its most bio-available form into the surrounding soil. This green manure is completely free of any of the pathogenic bacteria that comes from the intestines and feces of living creatures, such as E. coli. The Sinorhizobium meliloti (the parasitic soil organism, also known as Rhibozium) is the key to low cost organic farming on a commercial basis. Any threat to organic alfalfa is a threat to organic agriculture itself. As the super fine roots of alfalfa burrow through hardened soil, they break up and begin to absorb vital trace minerals that have been lost through topsoil erosion. Since these roots can travel as deep as a four story building rises high, they're able to access nutrients not available within the topsoil. It is at this time that the Rhibozium attaches itself and builds colonies that appear as nodules along the root system of alfalfa. These beneficial bacteria absorb nitrogen while alive and release it when decomposing. Some farmers purposefully bury the alfalfa through tilling and kill the plant thus killing the Rhibozium, which in turn releases massive amounts of nitrogen into the soil. Since alfalfa is a perennial, enough of the roots survive to insure next year's crop. However, being a perennial makes it far more vulnerable to cross-pollination by genetically modified alfalfa which has recently been approved by the U.S. Department of Agriculture. I would like to use this forum to sound the alarm once again by playing Paul Revere, and at the same time being accused of being Chicken Little by the skeptics that refuse to see what is right in front of their eyes. **Any threat to organic alfalfa is a direct assault on organic agriculture and it must be stopped!**

Just as Rachel Carson once sounded the alarm in *Silent Spring*, which finally woke America up to the cause and effect of DDT and other agricultural pesticides, today we need another movement to fight back against the paid experts who absolutely deny any risk from GMO's. Remember the fight is not over. While things did get better, (DDT was banned in the US) it is still used in Mexico and Turkey, which are both major food suppliers to the USA. Today the widespread use of chemicals that are still legal are still affecting indicator species which are especially vulnerable, particularly the pollinators like the honey bee, which farmers rely upon for the survival of oranges, grapefruits, apples and most flowering crops.

# COLONY COLLAPSE DISORDER

In the diverse and precariously balanced world of ecological systems, something as insignificant-looking as a bee could still carry the weight of a boulder and tip the scales towards a complete and catastrophic imbalance. That is what the world's food supply is facing at the moment with the advent of a phenomenon called Colony Collapse Disorder (CCD).

CCD is a phenomenon in which worker bees from a European honey-bee colony abruptly disappear. Bees abandoning their hives are commonplace enough and is a natural occurrence, but the drastic increase in rates of abandonment observed from the 1970's and peaking in 2006 has become a cause of alarm for agricultural experts. The impact of this phenomenon could be illustrated in the fact that the worth of global crops with honey-bees' pollination was estimated to be close to $200 billion in 2005 alone.

## SLEUTHING IN THE HIVE: SIGNS & SYMPTOMS OF CCD

An empty hive doesn't immediately equate to CCD. Certain conditions need to occur simultaneously for the abandonment to be classified as a CCD occurrence.

Presence of capped brood in abandoned colonies. (Bees normally will not abandon a hive until the capped brood have all hatched.)

Presence of food stores, both honey and bee pollen:

- Which are not immediately robbed by other bees, and

- Which when attacked by hive pests such as wax moth and small hive beetle, the attack is noticeably delayed.

- Persence of the queen bee: If the queen is not present, the hive died because it was queenless, which is not considered CCD.

Other signs that are a prelude to CCD are insufficient workforce to maintain the brood that is present and one that is mainly made up of young adult bees. The colony member may also show reluctance to consume provided feed before the collapse. A colony with a complete absence of adult bees with no or little build-up of dead bees in the hive, or in front of the hive is also a telltale sign of a collapsed colony.

## FINDING THE ANSWERS

Numerous studies have been undertaken to attempt to explain the mechanisms and causes of CCD in the hopes of finding a solution. It is the common scientific consensus that no single factor is causing CCD. Combinations of pesticides, mites, fungus, beekeeping practices, malnutrition, other pathogens, and immune-deficiencies are all possible culprits. Even so, certain pesticides called neonicotinoids are being singled out as especially harmful to the bees. Neonicotinoids are often used to prevent insects from destroying crops as early as at the time of planting, and could be carried within the plants and transferred to bees through pollen later in the growing season. Although not potent enough to kill the bees on contact, this kind of pesticide affects the overall health of bees and disrupts their homing systems, thus the absence of dead bodies inside the hive. The afflicted bees simply die away from their colonies.

## DAMAGE CONTROL

Neonicotinoids are currently banned in the European Union. Efforts to initiate a similar ban in the United States are also underway, and the Environmental Protection Agency is currently re-evaluating the pesticides.

The Mid-Atlantic Apiculture Research and Extension Consortium has also offered recommendations to beekeepers noticing the symptoms of CCD as early as 2007. Presently, new strains of bees that are more resistant to CCD culprits are being developed, especially in Europe where the campaign against CCD is more vigorous as their crops are more highly dependent on honey-bee pollination than those of the United States.

While the exact reason is debatable, what is undeniable is that entire colonies of bees have been dying off. For any number of reasons, some theorize that the chemicals used to discourage beetles and grubs from attacking the roots and flowers of certain crops have caused this crisis. Others believe it could be a parasitic mite. Regardless of whether it be climate change, herbicides, or GMO's, the impact on man is potentially life changing as common foods no longer become available without expensive hand or machine pollination.

Bees are not the only populations in danger of collapse, we need only look to see the rapid rise in birth defects as well as mental illness associated with aging, affecting the very youngest and eldest of our population, while an entire array of emerging viruses have begun to threaten all humans regardless of age. Whether it be Ebola, AIDS, SARS, Legionnaires' Disease, the bird flu, the swine flu or some other new strain of influenza, we are under siege and our immune systems are increasingly vulnerable. Drug resistant bacteria, flesh eating bacteria, and deadly mosquitos are now part of a new more dangerous world that is becoming less confident in our doctors' abilities to be our saviors.

This is all related. Just as we pour chemicals into the atmosphere and pollution into our oceans, we continue to increase the level of chemicals and pollutants in our bodies. The same crisis that is affecting the Earth, is affecting all of the creatures that inhabit it and we are not immune. In many ways our ignorance and arrogance has led to this crisis. But our intelligence, and our love for life and this planet can be the solution. It is time for each of us to begin to effectuate positive change in the world by changing our own lifestyle and our actions. When we begin to choose food for its ability to nourish our bodies and to keep us pure, then we will create a demand for pure and wholesome foods. That demand for pure and wholesome foods will create agriculture built around producing pure and wholesome crops which will create a pure and wholesome planet, and thus the very buying decisions of the inhabitance of this planet will dictate the future of the Earth and its ability to support them.

# THE EBOLA DILEMMA

The 2014 Ebola epidemic is by far the largest to occur in history, affecting multiple countries in West Africa and inciting a wave of paranoia across the globe. To date, there have been 19,065 reported cases, 7,388 of which led to death according to WHO statistics. Out of the 8 countries affected, 3 still remain as officially affected by the epidemic. These are Liberia, Sierra Leone, and Guinea. The outbreaks in Nigeria, Senegal, and Spain have already been declared over, after 42 days had elapsed since the last patient in isolation became laboratory negative for the disease.

The United States has also been touched by the outbreak when a Texan who had just arrived from Liberia tested positive for Ebola in September, 2014. Although the patient had succumbed to the disease, all his close contacts have been cleared as of November including 2 healthcare workers who had contracted the virus while caring for the patient. The third case was reported in New York when a medical aid worker who had arrived back from Guinea after serving with Doctors Without Borders was diagnosed with the disease. The patient has since recovered and given a clean bill of health as of November.

## WHAT ARE THE FACTS BEHIND THE FEARS?

Ebola, also known as Ebola hemorrhagic fever (EHF) or Ebola virus disease (EVD), is a rare and deadly disease caused by infection with one of the Ebola virus strains. Ebola can cause disease in humans and nonhuman primates such as monkeys, gorillas, and chimpanzees. EVD in humans is caused by four of five viruses of the genus Ebolavirus. The four are Bundibugyo virus (BDBV), Sudan virus (SUDV), Taï Forest virus (TAFV) and one simply called Ebola virus (EBOV, formerly Zaire Ebola virus). EBOV, species Zaire ebolavirus, is the most dangerous of the known EVD-causing viruses, and is responsible for the largest number of outbreaks. The fifth, Reston virus (RESTV), has caused disease in other primates but not in humans. The virus spreads by direct contact with blood or body fluids (including but not limited to urine, saliva, sweat, feces, vomit, breast milk, and semen) of an infected human or animal, and upon contact with a recently contaminated item or surface. The virus is able to survive on objects for a few hours in a dried state and can survive for a few days within body fluids. Semen and breast milk are believed to be capable of carrying the virus for several weeks to months.

In nature, fruit bats are thought to be the normal carrier of the virus, able to spread it without being affected by the disease.Symptoms may appear anywhere from 2 to 21 days after contamination, but the average is 8-10 days. These may generally include a fever that is usually higher than 38.3°C (100.9°F), severe headache, muscle pain that usually lasts even after recovery, weakness, fatigue, diarrhea, vomiting, abdominal pain, and unexplained bleeding or bruising.

The symptoms closely resemble that of other diseases such as influenza, malaria, cholera, typhoid fever, meningitis, and other viral hemorrhagic fevers. That is why it is of utmost importance for people who have come into close contact with confirmed EVD cases to have their blood samples tested for viral RNA, viral antibodies, or for the virus itself to confirm the diagnosis.

Recovery may begin between 7 and 14 days after the start of symptoms. Death, if it occurs, follows typically 6 to 16 days from the start of symptoms and is often due to low blood pressure from fluid loss.

No specific treatment or vaccine has been approved for Ebola, but survival rates increase with early supportive care consisting of rehydration and symptomatic treatment as well as the patient's immune response. Recovered patients develop antibodies that last for at least 10 years or even longer. It is not known if people who recover are immune for life or if they can become infected with a different species of Ebola.

The fact that there is no known cure yet for the disease, combined with its high mortality rate have fanned the growing paranoia even in countries untouched by the disease.

## CONCERNS ABOUT EBOLA AND FOOD SAFETY IN THE UNITED STATES

Although the CDC had been successful in the containment of the few Ebola cases in the US, concerns about the disease spreading through food products coming from affected countries have risen. Government health and food safety agencies have already released statements assuring the public that there has been no evidence of Ebola being spread by consuming food manufactured, grown, or imported from the affected countries. The only exception to this is bushmeat (meat from wild animals, such as monkeys or bats, hunted for food in developing regions of the world like some African countries). However, bringing in of bushmeat to the United States is illegal and authorities have already outlined strict guidelines to be enforced at all points of entry to prevent the introduction of bushmeat into the country.

# AIDS IN THE FACE OF OTHER GLOBAL PANDEMICS

As we approach halftime for this decade, global health desperately needs a timeout. Having been inundated by outbreaks of diseases such as cholera, measles, dengue fever, AH1N1, SARS, the dreaded Ebola virus, and more recently, the suspected bubonic and pneumonic plague threatening Madagascar, the world's populace could very well be turning hypochondriac.

These diseases which are highly communicable and brandish very high mortality rates is naturally panic-invoking and are able to easily grab the headlines. Despite this, there are still certain diseases that could never be pushed to the back of the shelves. One of these is AIDS.

## A BRIEF REVIEW

AIDS (acquired immune deficiency syndrome) is a disease spectrum of the human immune system caused by the human immunodeficiency virus (HIV). In medical parlance, AIDS pertains to the late stage symptoms of an infected person. The disease undermines the body's immune system, making the person more susceptible to common infections such as tuberculosis and other opportunistic infections and illnesses that don't usually affect people with healthy immune systems. During late stage infection the condition could be complicated by severe weight loss, a lung infection called pneumocystis pneumonia, Kaposi's sarcoma, or other AIDS-defining conditions.

The virus itself is transmitted primarily through unprotected sexual intercourse (including anal and oral sex), blood transfusions, hypodermic needles, and from mother to child during pregnancy, delivery or breastfeeding.

Although there have been numerous trials for cures and vaccines, none has been proven to be truly successful. As of the moment, the usual treatment after a suspected exposure to the virus consists of highly active antiretroviral therapy (HAART), which only slows the progression of the disease but doesn't eliminate the virus. For the most part, this is an expensive cocktail of drugs with numerous side effects. This has driven HIV patients to resort to alternative treatments such as micronutrient therapies to reduce mortality rates, and medical cannabis to alleviate symptoms, mostly without any sufficient medical evidence to their efficacy.

## NOT ENTIRELY OUT OF THE LIMELIGHT

Due to the disease's long incubating period that usually hinders early detection, AIDS has become more of a chronic rather than an acutely fatal disease around the globe, pushing it back from the headlines by more panic-inducing scourges like that of the Ebola and cholera outbreaks. This is understandable as the media is able to deliver blow by blow accounts of statistics rising and visual imagery of people literally dropping dead in a matter of days from infection. But looking at the bigger picture, AIDS is just as real, as frightening as any of them. Since the 60's, more than 30 million people had already succumbed to the disease worldwide and another 35 million is currently living with HIV/AIDS. Furthermore, AIDS is listed as the 6th leading cause of death in the world by WHO in a 2012 report.

On the brighter side though, a marked decrease in the number of HIV-related deaths between 2009 and 2012 has been attributed to the availability of antiretroviral therapy even in low- and middle-income regions.

Despite the fall in the number of people dying of AIDS, WHO has expressed dismay during the International AIDS Conference in July 2014, that the people most at risk of HIV are not getting the preventive health services they need. This, according to the international health entity, undermines the global progress on the HIV response. It enumerates men who have sexual intercourse with men, people in prison, injectable drug users, sex workers, and transgender people as some of the groups most at risk of infection yet are least likely to have access to HIV prevention, testing and treatment services due to discriminatory laws and policies in some countries. WHO released a consolidated guideline on HIV prevention, diagnosis, treatment and care for these key populations just before the conference, but admit that without the cooperation of countries with restrictive and discriminatory laws, the guidelines will have minimal impact. For example, in some countries discrimination is encouraged by laws and policies criminalizing sexual behaviors, drug use, gender expression, or perceived sexual orientation. Impacted individuals are unable to access the available health services for fear of being persecuted or stigmatized, opting to stay at a high risk of contracting the virus or silently bearing their symptoms if infected.

Though AIDS seems to be eclipsed nowadays by the more apocalyptic-like afflictions, it still remains a real and ever-present threat to many people worldwide. More than 12 million AIDS orphans and approximately 240 HIV-related deaths every hour could attest to the ferocity of this pandemic that has withstood medical advances for close to 4 decades already. The road towards a complete cure may still be long and unsure, but governments are being rallied to re-energize and reinforce HIV programs so that all key populations benefit from treatments and preventive advancements that are available now.

# BIRD FLU

Bird flu is the colloquial term for avian influenza, which refers to influenza caused by the *influenza A* virus that has adapted to birds. The term "bird flu" is similar to "swine flu," "horse flu," or "human flu" since it refers to an illness caused by any of the numerous different strains of the influenza A virus family that has adapted to a specific host. Adaptation is not exclusive though. Having adapted to one specific species does not preclude adaptations toward infecting a different species, but the virus strain may show preference or be highly pathogenic towards one species only.

The most highly pathogenic strain (H5N1) of the influenza A viruses had been spreading throughout Asia since 2003, but avian influenza only reached Europe in 2005 and the Middle East and Africa the year after. Companion birds in captivity and avian pets such as parrots are highly unlikely to contract the virus and the last reported case of a companion bird contracting the flu was in 2003. Pigeons are also not known to contract and spread the virus. Almost 84% of affected bird populations are composed of chicken and farm birds, while the remaining 15% are composed of wild birds.

## HITTING CLOSE TO HOME

The first human avian influenza A virus infection in North America was reported from Canada when a traveler who had recently returned from Beijing, China, was diagnosed as having contracted the H5N1 virus and died on January 3, 2014. This type of avian flu is endemic among poultry in that country as well as in Cambodia and Vietnam since 2003, and most of the 648 human cases of H5N1 infections occurred in people with direct or close contact with poultry in that region.

Although contracting H5N1 often results in serious illness with a very high mortality rate (60%), the spread of this virus from person to person is unlikely in the aforementioned case. The Centers for Disease Control and Prevention (CDC) considers that the health risks to people in North America posed by this single case is very low, but the agency will still disseminate information to clinicians in the United States about when and how to test for H5N1. Aside from this, the CDC is still working closely with Canadian public health partners and has offered support as needed. Another important measure that the CDC has secured for long-term preparedness against an H5N1 outbreak is the existence of a stockpile of H5N1 vaccine in the Strategic National Stockpile.

## PARANOIA OR PREPAREDNESS?

Concern over the H5N1 in Canada by the CDC is justifiable. Although the highly pathogenic avian influenza A has only been considered as endemic or ever present in poultry in at least six countries (Bangladesh, China, Egypt, India, Indonesia, and Vietnam) since 2003, and at the most sporadic in the rest of Asia, Europe, and Africa, the high mortality rate of the 648 laboratory-confirmed cases of human H5N1 infections is indeed concerning.

Furthermore, both human and avian influenza viruses evolve and swap genes frequently. If H5N1 or any other highly pathogenic strain of the influenza A virus would evolve the ability for efficient and sustained transmission among humans, an influenza pandemic could result with potentially devastating rates of illnesses and death worldwide. This is the primary factor moving not just the CDC, but international bodies like the World Health Organization (WHO) and Food and Agriculture Organization of the United Nations (FAO) to continue with routine surveillance of influenza viruses worldwide for changes that may have posed as risks to animal and public health.

One of the most fascinating facts about the bird and swine flu was revealed to me during my travels to Hong Kong, Taiwan and mainland China. I noticed first that their preferred meats were pork and duck, versus beef and chicken in the US, and that the pig farmers often raised ducks as well. It was there that I saw the beginnings of both the bird flu and the swine flu. You see as the ducks swim in the very water that the pigs drink from, they inevitably leave behind their feces as they defecate while swimming. Since the tropical temperatures create a warm environment that keep the bacteria in the feces alive, when the swine or pigs drink that water, they create the perfect environment to grow in their throats, where the fecal bacteria from the ducks mixes with the bacteria of the pig and begins to mutate. The pig's blood becomes infected through the stomach and ultimately the pigs become carriers of various parasites and viruses. When the pigs are taken to slaughter they are hung by their feet and their throats are slit. The blood rushes out and mixes with the virus which eventually infects the unsuspecting pig farmers who ultimately become carriers themselves. Through contact with their families and buyers at the market, they inevitably spread these new forms of viral infection. International travel and the popularity of outdoor markets where locals mix freely with tourists in turn become infected, and on their return trips home introduce these foreign flues to their local populations. It is ironic to think that most religious based food safety laws either forbid the consumption of pork, or the raising of pork and fowl together. So if the entire world ate a kosher or halal diet there would be none of the modern influenza epidemics as we know them.

## TEN DAY TRANSFORMATION

Beyond Green Food…

What started as a quest to save a nearly 900 lb. man from an obesity induced death, became a mission to save humanity from the siege of the latest plague (obesity), and the lessons learned became the genesis of my 10 day program to transform lives and break addiction to unhealthy food. A program that eventually became wildly popular in Hollywood and beyond and here is why…

"I only have 10 days to get ready for …". I hear it over and over. Every few months. Sometimes every few weeks. "I got your name from my (agent, manager, friend) and he/she said that you could get me in shape for my big (photo shoot, audition, pageant, fight, worldwide tour). I really need to get in shape fast! I need to lose weight without losing energy. I don't want to do anything dangerous or extreme, I just want to shed the pounds and look the best I've ever looked in my life." It seems like they always have less than two weeks. And sometimes, this is their big break, the opportunity that could change the course of their career. Now understand, most of these people could afford to go to any spa, any gym, any personal chef or nutritionist on the planet. They were coming to me specifically because of word-of-mouth recommendations from other industry insiders who had success with their own personal transformations.

The word throughout Hollywood was that there was something new, a "clean and green" way to lose weight and break food addictions. A program that no one else had. A simple way to transform your body in just 10 to 30 days. That's the origin of my Transformation Program and my 30-Day Transformation "Continuation Experience."

If they can do it, so can you.

Since I made my program available to the public, thousands and thousands of people have lost weight, re-set their metabolisms, broken their addictions to processed foods and cleansed their bodies. I believe that the 10-Day Transformation is the fastest, healthiest, simplest, least expensive way to lose weight and keep it off for life. But the weight loss is just a healthy side effect of the reboot of your metabolism. More importantly, we have seen people transition from short-term results into long-term lifestyle changes that are based on clean and green eating.

The concept behind my program is really quite simple. I use nutrient-dense superfoods, slow-burning carbs and highly-digestible protein. All vegan. All natural. More important, you will not be consuming ANY processed, irradiated, denatured, artificial or genetically-modified ingredients. This is anabolic eating, so you won't be sacrificing your long-term health for short-term results. Your body will love it! I guarantee it.

I discovered that losing 5-20 pounds is easy, once you learn to give the body what it needs. On my program you will create total cellular satisfaction, support anabolic muscle building and infuse the body with cellular defense foods.

# GENERAL RECOMMENDATIONS

- Select foods that are organic or as close to the earth as possible.

- Eat slowly and chew your food well - 30 chews per mouthful.

- Eat until you are 80% full as satiety signals take time to register.

- Be thankful & appreciate the food that nourishes you.

Below are some of my favorite foods.

Some of My Favorite Protein Sources

1. 1 or 2 eggs hardboiled, poached or fried in coconut oil. (Choose eggs from free-roaming chickens that eat grass and insects and have high omega 3 fat content.)

2. 1/2 cup organic cottage cheese, (great when you add purple grapes).

3. 1 serving of free-range chicken (from free-roaming chickens that eat grass and insects and have high omega 3 fat content).

4. 1 serving (3-4 ounces) of Wild salmon (preferably line-caught salmon vs. farmed salmon which does not have all of the nutrients and essential fats).

5. 1 cup (cooked) lentils or other legumes, except soy.

6. 1/4 cup hummus (beans, tahini, spices and olive oil – the quality of the olive oil will determine the quality of the hummus).

7. 2 cups broccoli (cooked or uncooked, raw or lightly steamed is best).

8. 2 tbsp. natural almond, sunflower or sesame butter (no high fructose corn syrup – should be just the nuts, one possible exception is "sea salt").

9. Pinto, navy, lima or other beans. I recommend fava beans for those who are concerned with Parkinson's as fava beans are a great source of "l-dopa".

10. Purium's Vegan Protein Options (Spirulina, Master Aminos, L.O.V.E. Super Meal)

Tips for protein:

- Protein is best consumed in the morning when we have high levels of HCL.

- Meat should always be combined with green vegetables to reduce the impact of its toxins.

- Avoid the burnt crispy parts of meat as they are carcinogenic.

- Eat grass-fed beef, free-roaming chicken and wild caught salmon as they are the highest quality in their category.

- Don't combine meat with carbohydrates or sugars (i.e. bread, soda, fruits).

- Consume no more than 6 oz. of animal flesh in any 24 hour period to avoid creating uric acid and harming your kidneys.

Some of My Favorite Complex Carbohydrates:

1. 3/4 cup cooked red, black or brown rice.

2. 3/4 cup quinoa.

3. 3/4 cup couscous.

4. 2 slices sprouted grain bread.

5. 2 medium size buckwheat or whole grain pancakes or waffles.

6. Purple or sweet potatoes (approximately the size of your fist).

7. 1 serving of whole grain breakfast cereal (without artificial ingredients, colors or preservatives).

8. Sprouted grain or veggie pastas (without artificial ingredients, colors or preservatives).

9. Oatmeal, cream of buckwheat or other whole grain hot cereal (without artificial ingredients, colors or preservatives).

10. Purium's Activated Barley

Tips for Complex Carbs:

- "Crack" rice by stirring in hot pan to release protein before cooking.

- Buy organic grains whenever possible.

- Buckwheat and Activated Barley pancakes create great glucose control.

- Purple potatoes help your body like blueberries.

- Try spaghetti squash as an alternative to pasta.

Some of My Favorite Fruit:

1. Cherries (the darker the better).

2. Blueberries (wild if possible).

3. Plums (the smaller the better).

4. Raspberries/blackberries/mulberries, etc. (best to get organic, difficult to wash and often full of pesticides otherwise).

5. Apples (a more unique variety is best).

6. Peppers (delicious when stuffed with avocado or hummus and rice, may also add a lean protein source such as chicken).

7. Watermelon and other melons (best eaten alone).

8. Avocados (yes, it is a fruit! Amazing spread for toast, or as guacamole or simply by itself).

9. Cucumbers (make them into chips - slice and squeeze fresh lemon, cayenne and sea salt).

10. Tomatoes (yes, also a fruit! Try to get heirloom whenever possible).

11. Almonds (yes, also a fruit as well!).

12. Papaya.

13. Purple Grapes.

Tips for Fruit:

- Eat organic or wash well – pay attention to the current "Dirty Dozen" list which tells you the fruits and veggies to absolutely avoid buying non-organic that year.

- Eat fruit before other food and never right after, there is one exception for not having fruit with other items - cottage cheese and fruit do go well together.

- Avoid white and green grapes.

- Don't mix melons with other fruit.

- Eat apples in the morning to help wake you up as a coffee alternative.

- Don't remove the skin because the most nutrients are contained there (exceptions are bananas, oranges, mangos, avocados and melons, etc. – use your best judgment).

- Dried fruit should be eaten separately.

Some of My Favorite Veggies:

1. Kale (best marinated or steamed).

2. Broccoli (use as crudités, sautéed or for a high protein omelet.

3. Cabbage (great in slaws, soups and sauerkraut).

4. Squash (delicious when sautéed with red bell pepper, red onion, and garlic in coconut oil or organic butter).

5. Asparagus.

6. Mushrooms (great immune boosters).

7. Carrots.

8. Sea Vegetables (wakame, hijiki, dulse - use in soups, dips, sauces and salads).

9. Celery (crudités dipped in hummus or nut butter or another healthy dipping sauce, amazing base for any soup).

10. Cilantro and parsley (not just for garnish – great for digestion and deodorizing breath, also great in pesto).

Tips for Veggies:

- Eat as many brightly colored veggies as possible.

- Steamed is okay but do not overcook.

- Sauté in organic butter, olive oil or coconut oil.

- Eat raw veggies with hummus or guacamole.

- Marinate raw veggies for better flavor.

My Recommended Liquids:

1. Spring water w/lemon.

2. Cranberry, pomegranate, hibiscus juice.

3. Aloe vera juice .

4. Coconut water.

5. Unfiltered apple or prune juice with lots of fiber.

6. Orange juice or grapefruit juice with lots of pulp.

7. Kefir, Kombucha.

8. Green Tea.

9. Concord grape juice.

10. Pineapple juice.

Tips for Liquids:

- Drink room temperature in the morning to help flush kidneys (warm water is easier on digestion).

- Squeeze lemon in your water to increase its alkalizing ability.

- Use unsweetened cranberry juice to fight urinary tract infections.

- Drink Hibiscus tea to reduce sugar cravings.

- Use aloe vera to fight ulcers.

- Coconut water is the ultimate sports replenishment drink.

- Drink raw apple juice to fight kidney stones and gout.

- Prune juice relieves constipation.

Some of My Favorite Cooking & Salad Oils:

1. Organic Coconut Oil

2. Organic Raw Butter

3. Grapeseed Oil

4. Safflower Oil

5. Macadamia Nut Oil

6. Avocado Oil

7. Extra Virgin Olive Oil

8. Green Tea Seed Oil

9.  Red Palm Oil

10. Sunflower Seed Oil

Tips for cooking and prepping with fats:

- High Heat (Green Tea Seed, Grapeseed, Avocado, Macadamia).

- Medium High Heat (Coconut, Red Palm, Safflower).

- Sauté / Low Heat (Butter, Olive Oil, Sunflower).

- Consume 1 tsp. of raw coconut oil daily for general health.

## FOOD

Eat more brightly colored fruits and vegetables. Do not eat foods with artificial colors since they could be harmful. Eat more healthy fats from flaxseeds, avocados, chia seeds, coconuts, rice bran, and/or oily, wild caught fish. Avoid all trans-fats, hydrogenated oils, partially hydrogenated oils, soybean oils, and reduce animal fat. Eat more high fiber and gluten free whole grains, seeds, legumes and bran. Avoid white flour, white rice, and any processed/denatured, fortified grain product. Consume wild or free roaming grass fed protein and/or preferably substitute high quality vegan and vegetarian protein options as often as possible. Avoid commercially produced animals, farmed fish, cured meat, and animals treated with antibiotics and hormones.

## WATER

Be sure to drink 1/2 your body weight in ounces per day. It is very important to keep your body hydrated. During the fast you can consume up to your body weight in ounces of water each day. If you are properly hydrated, you should urinate every 2-3 hours during the daytime.

## EXERCISE

Stress is stress. Too much exercise is like too many calories, we recommend 45 minutes to an hour, 4 times a week (except during the 10 Day Transformation).

Make sure you sweat, allow time for warm-up and cool-down, and focus on core workouts and cardio. Simply be active, take the stairs, carry your groceries, play with the kids, go dancing, and be sure to have fun.

## SLEEP

We recommend 7-8 hours but getting enough deep sleep is the key, 2 hours of deep sleep per night is ideal since 80% of repair and detoxification are triggered during this time. Deficiencies of melatonin and trace minerals contribute to poor sleep.

## MORE FROM DAVID

Stretch and take 3 deep breaths upon waking. Take care of your teeth. Get 40 minutes of direct sunlight daily. Accept change. Find peace with what you do not know. Face your fears. Breathe consciously. Express your emotions. Laugh, cry and smile. Love without condition. Accept that you are worthy of being loved. Inspire a child. Learn to heal yourself. Take joy in giving. Be flexible in your body and in your mind. Forgive yourself and others easily. Stimulate your mind. Stay busy and have a purpose. Discover that the greatest joys can come from the smallest things.

Make the world better because you were here.

- David Sandoval

## IN CONCLUSION

In my study of foods, their energies, and how they contribute to our physiological well-being, I have come to emphasize the life force or *chi* energy. It transcends any knowledge we have regarding nutrients or phytochemicals and relates directly to the living energy that is part of all green plants.

Each of these scientists has furthered the work of their predecessors. I hope that in my own small way, I can make my own contribution to the understanding of the gifts Nature offers us, and why they are so incredibly valuable to humanity. I want to encourage everyone to embrace the healing miracle of green foods.

# RESOURCES

## OASIS RETREAT

One of my inspirations, Anne Wigmore, created Hippocrates Health Institute near Boston, MA, to allow people a place to go to de-stress, to learn to heal and to grow. Another one of my mentors, Bernard Jensen, also created a similar space in California where he taught his passion--iridology and naturopathy. They were the inspiration for what is today both my home and my sacred ground. It is my legacy, my own healing center with over a dozen rooms, half a dozen authentic Sioux Lakota teepees and abundant ways to spend leisure and learning time. I call it the Native Springs Oasis.

But it did not start that way. It started when I wanted to find ideal, virgin, high-country farmland that met my requirements. That meant it needed to be at least 100 miles away from any polluting industry, it had to have rich valley soil surrounded by 8000 ft. peeks, and pure local water for irrigation. I found it, so I bought it and set about planning. Unfortunately, my dreams of large scale organic farming were denied when the local neighbors preferred the quiet bucolic setting, and objected to the local city council. However, with every ending emerges a new beginning. And the Oasis was born.

When I first set out to create this space, my infrastructures were few but the requests began to come in. Our first group included 18 women each suffering from various forms and in various stages of breast cancer. The time we spent talking about their fear, their anger, their hope, their families, their past and their now much uncertain futures was life changing. It set the stage for many healing retreats to come, but none could ever move me the way that first one did. I often think about those women and where they are today.

Perhaps the single most interesting guest at the oasis was Manny "Tiny' Yarbrough, once listed in the Guinness Book of World Records as the largest athlete in history. This six foot eight inch tall, 650 pound sumo champion had enjoyed the limelight as a guest on The Letterman Show, Jay Leno, Jimmy Kimmel, Jimmy Fallon, Good Morning America, and many others as an American Hero. After a series of personal crises, he had ballooned up and out of control to an astounding 880 lbs., and was facing an uncertain future with an unstable body. He was racked with diabetes, sleep apnea, high blood pressure, osteoarthritis, and a number of other major and minor ailments that left him bed ridden and near death. We brought him to the Oasis, and after a few short weeks of superfood infused shakes and concentrated vegan proteins, combined with water aerobics and good old fashion love, he managed to lose over 260 lbs., and was hovering at (a much healthier for him) 600 lbs. in just 5 months.

Our next high level visitor, Colum Best, son of perhaps the greatest footballer in European history, and a famous Hollywood playboy. He was caught in a compromising position by the tabloids as Lindsey Lohan's love interest. Challenged to clean up his act in 40 days of sobriety and celibacy by MTV Europe, the Oasis was chosen as a safe get-away from temptation.

The breathtaking and picturesque setting of the Native Springs Oasis has also attracted Hollywood's attention. One of my best times at the Oasis was when we put together a group of aspiring actors, actresses, directors, producers, writers and musicians with camera and support crew to participate in the 48 hr. Film Festival for the very first time. The creative and talented ensemble soon went to work and produced a short film for the ages. It was nominated for six awards, unprecedented in festival history, and took home one. Also, a first for a maiden voyage. Since then other Hollywood inspired films and shoots have taken place here, as have music videos, Shaman ceremonies, and celebrity birthdays and weddings! We have also had some of the liveliest music festivals with high level entertainment, and 24 hr. fun.

I have to say my favorite groups are the groups that come to learn about my latest programs and products which I call detoxifications, an amazing combination of off-sight outing, on-sight fun, and delicious, nutritious food preparation and instruction. We now hold P.H.P. academies and offer certified training courses in weight management, sports nutrition, detoxification, and anti-aging. When not learning, we are seeking adventures… whether we are visiting the amazing sequoias, (among the oldest and tallest trees on the planet) kayaking down class 5 rapids, or cruising in an inner tube down a lazy river there is always fun to be found. We have a one mile novice hiking/jogging trail, and a 3.5 mile, 3500 foot climb we call the horse shoe that has been navigated by the fittest man in Hawaii, champion Ikaika Pascua, in a mind boggling 35 minutes. I personally love taking people to the hot springs located along a raging river, a short quarter mile hike that is worth the effort.

Local native points of interest include Red Rock Canyon, where the visitor information center includes a native elder, and the Hui Nui Trading Post, located on the shores of Lake Isabella. Perhaps the most interesting native ruins lay right on this land itself and are worthy of a short hike from your room where you can delicately examine the circle of elders fire pit, the gathering of tribes adobe building and even see an authentic Native American rock fort. In honor of this land's native heritage, we have built our own teepee village that currently offers 5 – 18 foot diameter family style teepees, and 1 – 28 foot diameter grand meeting teepee, that are often used for massages, ceremonies, camping, and temporary trading posts.

Some of the favorite man made activities, include our far infrared sauna (FIS), our intimate yoga room, our bamboo jacuzzi garden, our 200 ft. long water slide, two 75 ft. zip lines, and water volley ball in our aerobics pool. Guests enjoy picking fresh veggies from our chili garden and preparing meals together in our over-sized family kitchen.

Our efforts at growing watermelons became a feeding frenzy for our local uninvited, but welcome guests, including bears, coyotes, mountain lions, birds, foxes, rabbits, and road runners. These animals all flock to this area, since it is truly an Oasis in the desert.

The Oasis is also designated riparian habitat, meaning it is vital to the reproductive efforts and survival of endangered and protected species of birds. In addition to wood ducks, we are blessed to be visited by over 37 varieties of migrating and local avian life.

In the future, we envision adding mud baths, obstacle courses, bigger and longer zip lines, slack lines, a game room, a muscle beach type workout area and even kayaking runs on my stream. We want to teach small scale organic farming and survival techniques, as well as host study groups, seminars, summits, retreats and music festivals.

Our dedication to being green includes a vision to be completely off of the grid, have all composting toilets, a functioning grey water system, and to showcase multiple green (non-polluting) energy sources, and build the modal for a high tech, low tech fusion lifestyle.

The Oasis Retreat is located three hours north of Los Angeles, near beautiful Lake Isabella in Kern County, California. This serene 160 acre ranch is the ideal setting for one to detoxify and rejuvenate. Visitors can enjoy nature walks along our "Living Water" creek fed by nearly 100 artesian springs, or choose to bask in the sun near the 28,000 gallon fresh water pool, then spend nights gazing into the starlit skies.

Adding a nice touch to the secluded culture of Oasis Retreat, each room has its own private bath and private entrance. The country-style setting of the Oasis Retreat allows for individuals, families or groups to enjoy the outdoors as Mother Nature intended. Take a break from cell phones, cable TV and the hectic lifestyle associated with city living. The holistic-oriented staff leads yoga, performs massage therapy, provides your daily regimen of nutritional supplements, prepares living and vegetarian meals, builds bonfires and hosts daily activities. Join us at the Oasis Retreat for an experience of a lifetime!

*"I wanted the Oasis to be a sanctuary away from the stress that most people experience in their lives. A place of transition where one can reflect on what would be necessary to heal physically, emotionally and spiritually, and take positive steps toward this new life. The Oasis Retreat is a place to learn routines that can be taken home to help ensure you accomplish your goals."* —David Sandoval

## OASIS RETREAT

3135 Kelso Valley Road, Weldon, CA 93283. For more information or to make a reservation, please email trydavesway@gmail.com.

# REFERENCES

## CHAPTER 1

"Agriculture: origins," http://www.primalseeds.org/agricult.htm Martin, Angus, and Wadley, Greg, "The origins of agriculture – a biological perspective and a new hypothesis," *Australian Biologist* 6: 96 – 105, June 1993, posted at http://www.vegan-straight- edge.org.uk/GW_paper.htm

"Hunter-Gatherers.org: Facts and Theories About Hunter-Gatherers." http://hunter-gatherers.org/facts-and-theories.html

Stables GJ, et al, "Changes in vegetables and fruit consumption and awareness among US adults: results of the 1991 and 1997 5 a day for better health program surveys," *J Am Dietetic Assoc* 2002;102:809-817.

## CHAPTER 2

Dingley KH, et al, "Effect of dietary constituents with chemopreventive potential on adduct formation of a low dose of the heterocyclic amines PhIP and IQ and phase II hepatic enzymes," *Nutr Cancer* 2003;46(2):212-21.

Ferruzzi MG, Failla ML, Schwartz SJ, "Sodium copper chlorophyllin: in vitro digestive stability and accumulation by Caco-2 human intestinal cells," *J Agric Food Chem* 2002 Mar 27;50(7):2173-9.

Guo D, et al, "Inhibition by chlorophyllin of 2-amino-3-methylinidazo-[4,5-f]quinolone-induced tumorigenesis in the male F344 rat," *Cancer Letters* 1995 Aug 16;195(1-2):161-5.

Mercola J, "Chlorophyll is not the same as hemoglobin," http://www.mercola.com/2002/mar/23/chlorophyll_hemoglobin.htm

Natsume Y, et al, "Assessment system for dioxin absorption in the small intestine and prevention of its absorption by food factors," *Biofactors* 2004;21(1-4):375-7.

Schoenhals K, "Green power: superfoods that really pack a punch; chlorella growth factor; green Superfoods," *Better Nutrition* October 1, 2004.

deVogel J, et al, "Green vegetables, red meat and colon cancer: chlorophyll prevents the cytotoxic and hyperproliferative effects in rat colon," *Carcinogenesis* 2005 Feb;26(2):387-93.

## CHAPTER 3

Chen TS, Chen PS, "Intestinal autointoxication: a medical leitmotif," *J Clin Gastroenterol* 1989 Aug;11(4):434-41.

"Enzymes and longevity," www.living-foods.com/articles/enzymes.html Fahey JW, "Antioxidant functions of sulforaphane: a potent inducer of Phase II detoxication enzymes," *Food Chem Toxicol* 1999 Sep-Oct;37(9-10):973-9. Gots RE, "Medical hypothesis and medical practice: autointoxication and multiple chemical sensitivities," *Regul Toxicol Pharmacol* 1993 Aug;18(1)2-12.

Grant AM, et al, "Oral vitamin D3 and calcium for secondary prevention of low-trauma fractures in elderly people: randomized evaluation of calcium or vitamin D, a randomized placebo-controlled trial," *Lancet* 2005, May 7-13;365(9471):1621-8.

Jacobs EI, White E, "Constipation, laxative use, and colon cancer among middle-aged adults," *Epidemiology* 1998 Jul;9(4):385-91.

National Health and Nutrition Examination Survey (NHANES) Newell KJ, Tannock IF, "Reduction of intracellular pH as a possible mechanism for killing cells in acidic regions of solid tumors: effects of carbonylcyanide-3-chlorophenylhydrazone," *Cancer Res* 1989 Aug 15;49(16):4477-82.

Porthouse J, et al, "Randomized controlled trial of calcium and supplementation with cholcalciferol (vitamin D3) for prevention of fractures in primary care," *British Medical Journal* 2005 Apr 30;330(7498):1003.

Roberts MC, et al, "Constipation, laxative use, and colon cancer in a North Carolina population," *American Journal of Gastroenterology* 2003 Apr;98(4):857-64.www.agingsociety.net

## CHAPTER 4

Ben-Arye E, et al, "Wheatgrass juice in the treatment of active distal ulcerative colitis," *Scandinavian Journal of Gastroenterology* 2002;37(4):444-449.

Flohe L, "Superoxide dismutate for therapeutic use: clinical experience, dead ends and hopes," *Molecular and Cellular Biochemistry* 1988 Dec;84(2):123- 31.

"Grass," http://www.infoplease.com/ce6/sci/A0821581.html, accessed 11/4/2005.

Regan E, et al, "Extracellular superoxide dismutase and oxidant damage in osteoarthritis," *Arthritis and Rheumatism* 2005 Nov;52(11):3479-91.

Schnabel CF, "Verdict from a Guinea Pig Jury after 12 weeks deliberation," *Acres USA*, 1973.

St.Clair D, et al, "Modulation of skin tumorigenesis by superoxide dismutase," *Biomed Pharmacother* 2005 May;59(4):209-14.

## CHAPTER 5

Banu SM, Selvendiran K, Singh JP, Sakthisekaran D, "Protective effect of Emblica officinalis ethanolic extract against 7,12-dimethylbenz(a) anthracene (DMBA) induced genotoxicity in Swiss albino mice," *Hum Exp Toxicol* 2004 Nov;23(11):527-31.

Bhattacharya A, Ghosal S, Bhattacharya SK, "Antioxidant activity of tannoid principles of Emblica officinalis (amla) in chronic stress-induced changes in rat brain," *Indian J Exp Biol* 2000 Sep;38(9):877-80.

Carlucci MJ, et al, "Antiherpetic activity and mode of action of natural carrageenans of diverse structural types," *Antiviral Res* 1999 Sep;43(2):93-102.

Carlucci MJ, et al, "Antiherpetic and anticoagulant properties of carrageenans from the red seaweed Gigartina skottsbergii and their cyclized derivatives: correlation between structure and biological activity," *Int J Biol Macromol* 1997 Apr;20(2):97-105.

Carlucci MJ, et al, "Inhibitory action of natural carrageenans on Herpes simplex virus infection of mouse astrocytes," *Chemotherapy* 1999 Nov-Dec;45(6):429-36

Carlucci MJ, et al, "Protective effect of a natural carrageenan on genital herpes simplex virus in mice," *Antiviral Res* 2004 Nov;64(2):137-41.

Cheng JY, Shih MF, "Improving glycogenesis in streptozocin (STZ) diabetic mice after administration of green algae Chlorella," *Life Sci* 2006 Feb 9;78(11):1181-6.

Dalton LW, "Controversy: viral invasions," *Chemical & Engineering News*, 2004 May 24;82(21):45-53. Posted at http://pubs.acs.org/cen/coverstory/8221/8221viral.html Accessed 3/17/06

Hirahashi T, et al, "Activation of the human innate immune system by Spirulina: augmentation of interferon production and NK cytotoxicity by oral administration of hot water extract of Spirulina platensis," *Int Immunopharmacol* 2002;2:423-34.

Konishi F, et al, "Enhanced resistance against *Escherichia coli* infection by subcutaneous administration of the hot-water extract of *Chlorella vulgaris* in cyclophosphamide-treated mice," *Cancer Immunol Immunother* 1990;32(1):1-7.

Mason R, M.S., "Chlorella and Spirulina: Green Supplements for Balancing the Body," *Alternative and Complementary Therapies* 2001 June; 7(3):161- 165.

Morita K, et al, "Chlorella accelerates dioxin excretion in rats," *J Nutr* 1999;129(9):1731-36.

Perianayagam JB, et al, "Evaluation of anti-pyretic and analgesic activity of Emblica officinalis Gaertn," *J Ethnopharmacol* 2004 Nov;95(1):83-5.

Pore RS, "Detoxification of chlordecone poisoned rats with chlorella and chlorella-derived sporopollenin," *Drug Chem Toxicol 1*984;7(1):57-71.

Rao TP, Sakaguchi N, Juneja LR, Wada E, Yokozawa T, "Amla (Emblica of-fici- nalis Gaertn.) extracts reduce oxidative stress in streptozotocin-induced diabetic rats," *J Med Food* 2005 Fall;8(3):362-8.

Sai Ram M, Neetu D, Deepti P, Vandana M, Ilavazhagan G, Kumar D, Sel-vamurthy W, "Cytoprotective activity of Amla (Emblica officinalis) against chromium (VI) induced oxidative injury in murine macrophages," *Phytother Res* 2003 Apr;17(4):430-3.

Sancheti G, et al, "Chemopreventive action of emblica officinalis on skin carcinogenesis in mice," *Asian Pac J Cancer Prev* 2005 Apr-Jun;6(2):197- 201.

Singh I, et al, "Radioprotection of Swiss albino mice by Emblica officinalis," *Phytother Res* 2005 May;19(5):444-6.

Sultana S, et al, "Effect of Emblica officinalis (Gaertn) on CCI4 induced hepatic toxicity and DNA synthesis in Wistar rats," *Indian J Exp Biol* 2005 May;43(5):430-6.

Sultana S, et al, "Emblica officinalis reverses thioacetamide-induced oxida-tive stress and early promotional events of primary hepatocarcinogenesis," *J Pharm Pharmacol* 2004 Dec;56(12):1573-9.

Tanaka K, Tomita Y, Tsuruta M, et al, "Oral administration of Chlorella vulgaris augments concomitant antitumor immunity," *Immunopharmacol Immunotoxicol* 1990;12(2):277-91

Tasduq SA, et al, "Reversal of fibrogenic events in liver by Emblica officinalis (fruit), an Indian natural drug," *Biol Pharm Bull* 2005 Jul;28(7):1304-6.

## CHAPTER 6

Adachi N, et al, "(-)-Epigallocatechin gallate attenuates acute stress responses through GABAergic system in the brain," *Eur J Pharmacol* 2006 Jan 31.

Baliga MS, Katiyar SK, "Chemoprevention of photocarcinogenesis by selected dietary botanicals," *Photochem Photobiol Sci* 2006 Feb;5(2):243-53.

Bastianetto S, et al, "Neuroprotective effects of green and black teas and their catechin gallate esters against beta-amyloid-induced toxicity," *Eur J Neurosci* 2006 Jan;23(1):55-64.

Funahashi H, et al, "Seaweed prevents breast cancer?" *Jpn J Cancer Res* 2001 May;92(5):483-7.

Mandel S, et al, "Green tea catechins as brain-permeable, natural ion chelators-antioxidants for the treatment of neurodegenerative disorders," *Mol Nutr Food Res* 2006 Feb;50(2):229-34.

Na HK, Surh YJ, "Intracellular signaling network as a prime chemopreventive target of −(-) epigallocatechin gallate," *Mol Nutr Food Res* 2006 Feb;50(2):159-2.

Shimizu M, et al, "EGCG inhibits activation of HER3 and expression of cyclooxygenase-2 in human colon cancer cells," *J Exp Ther Oncol* 2005;5(1):69-78.

Stangl V, Lorenz M, Stangl K, "The role of tea and tea flavonoids in cardiovas- cular health," *Mol Nutr Food Res* 2006 Feb;50(2):208-28.

"Substance from green leaves dampens appetite," Physorg.com, http://www.physorg.com/news70112308.html , accessed 6/30/06.

Suzuki N, et al, "Antioxidative activity of animal and vegetable dietary fibers," *Biofactors* 2004;21(1-4):329-33.

Wolfram S, Wang Y, Thielecke F, "Antiobesity effects of green tea: from bedside to bench," *Mol Nutr Food Res* 2006 Feb;50(2):176-87.

## CHAPTER 7

Maruyama H, Watanabe K, Yamamoto I, "Effect of dietary kelp on lipid peroxidation and glutathione peroxidase activity in livers of rats given breast carcinogen DMBA," *Nutr Cancer* 1991;15(3-4):221-8.

Sakakibara H, et al, "Effects of Japanese kelp (kombu) on life span of benzo[a]pyrene-fed mice," *J Nutr Sci Vitaminol* (Tokyo) 2005 Oct;51(5):369-73.

## CHAPTER 8

Aoi W, Naito Y, Sakuma K, Kuchide M, Tokuda H, Maoka T, Toyokuni S, Oka S, Yasuhara M, Yoshikawa T. (2003). Astaxanthin limits exercise-induced skeletal and cardiac muscle damage in mice. Antioxid Redox Signal, 5(1):139-144.

Aoi W, Naito Y, Takanami Y, Ishii T, Kawai Y, Akagiri S, Kato Y, Osawa T, Yoshikawa T. (2008). Astaxanthin improves muscle lipid metabolism in exercise via inhibitory effect of oxidative CPT I modification. Biochem. Biophys. Res. Com., 366:892–897.

Arad, Shoshana. Microalgal Ointment for Treating Herpes, Ben-Gurion University of the Negev, Israel, 2000.

Cole and Sheath, (Ed.) Biology of the Red Algae, Cambridge University Press, Cambridge, 1990.

Dieg et al. "Development of dermal lesions in adult mice infected with *Herpes simplex* virus:simplexevelopment of dermal lesions in adult mice infected with ress, Cambridge, 1990. ffect of oxidative CPT I modification. Biochem. Biophys. Res. Com., 366:892le damage in m

Dieg et al. "Evaluation of extracts of marine algae for antiviral activity in experimental *Herpes simplex* infections of infant mice." In 52nd Technical Progress Report, Section 4, Naval Biosciences Laboratory, School of Public Health, University of California, Berkeley, 1977.

Dieg et al. "Inhibition of herpes virus replication by marine algae extracts." Anitimicrb. Ag. Chemother 6:524-525, 1974.

Douglas et al. "Acyclovir and Genital Herpes." N Eng J of Medicine, Vol. 310 No. 24, 1551-56, 1984.

Ehresmann et al. "Antiviral properties of algal polysaccharides and related compounds," in H.A. Hoppe et al. (ed.), Marine Algae in Pharmaceutical Science, W. de Gruyter, NY, 293-302, 1979.

Ehresmann et al. "Antiviral substances from California marine algae." J. Phycol. 13:37-40, 1979.

Fukamauchi, M. (2007). Food functionality of astaxanthin-10: Synergistic effects of astaxanthin-10 intake and aerobic exercise. Food Style 21, 11(10). [In Japanese]

Gonzales et al. «Polysaccharides as antiviral agents: onzales et al. «Polysaccharides as antiviral agents:f astaxanthin-10 intake and aerobic ex- ercis

Hatch et al. "Chemical characterization and therapeutic evaluation of an- ti-Herpes-virus polysaccharides from species of Dumontiaceae," in H. A. Hoppe et al. (ed.), Marine Algae in Pharmaceutical Science, W. de Gruyter, NY, 346-363, 1979.

Ikeuchi M, Koyama T, Takahashi J, Yazawa K. (2006). Effects of astaxan- thin supplementation on exercise-induced fatigue in mice. Bio. Pharm. Bull., 29(10):2106-2110.

Lee SJ, Bai SK, Lee KS, Namkoong S, Na HJ, Ha KS, Han JA, Yim SV, Chang K, Kwon YG, Lee SK, Kim YM. (2003). Astaxanthin Inhibits Nitric Oxide Production and Inflammatory Gene Expression by Suppressing IkB

Kinase-dependent NF-kB Activation. Mol. Cells, 16(1):97-105.

Malmsten C, Lignell A. (2008). Dietary supplementation with astaxanthin rich algal meal improves muscle endurance – a double blind study on male students. Carotenoid Science 13:20-22.

Mitsuya et al. "Dextran sulfate suppression of viruses in the HIV family: Inhibition of virion binding to CD4 and cells." Science 240:646-649, 1988.

Nakashima et al. "Antiretroviral activity in a marine red alga: Reverse transcriptase inhibition by an aqueous extract of Schizymenia pacifica." Journal Cancer Res. Clin Oncol 113:413-16, 1987.

Neushul. "Antiviral carbohydrates from marine red algae." Hydrobiologia 204/205:99-104, 1990.

Pitchford, Paul. Healing with Whole Foods. North Atlantic Books, Berkeley, California, 1993.

Richards et al. "Antiviral activity of extracts from marine algae." Antimicrob. Agents Chemother. 14:24-30, 1978.

Sawaki K, Yoshigi H, Aoki K, Koikawa N, Azumane A, Kaneko K, Yamaguchi M. (2002). Sports performance benefits from taking natural astaxanthin characterized by visual activity and muscle fatigue improvements in humans. J Clin.Therap. Med., 18(9):73-88.

Serkedjieva, J. "Antiherpes virus effect of the red marine alga *Polysiphonia denudata*." *Z naturforsch* [C], 2000;55(9-10):830-835.

Straus et al., "Suppression of frequently recurring genital herpes." N Eng J of Medicine, Vol 310, No. 24, 1984.

Thomson and Fowler. "Carrageenan: A review of its effects on the immune system: Agents and Actions," 11:265-273, 1981.

**Patent**

Medicament for improvement of duration of muscle function or treatment of muscle disorders or diseases. US # 6,245,818, WO9911251.

# CHAPTER 9

*The Essene Gospel of Peace. Book Four. The Teachings of the Elect.* Translated and edited by Edmond Bordeaux Szekely, International Biogenic Society, 1981.

# INDEX

ACNE, 20, 25, 27, 121, 137, SEE ALSO SKIN HEALTH

AGING/ANTI-AGING, 19, 39, 49, 79, 90, 129, 208

AIDS, 20, 177, 190, 191, 192, SEE ALSO HIV

ALGAE, 8, 9, 11, 35, 79, 87, 98, 99, 100, 130, 135, 136, 143, 144
      RED MARINE, 101, 138, 147, 148, 149, 150, 151, 152

ALLERGIES, 17, 18, 27, 47, 54, 65, 79, 101, 142

ALOE VERA, 94, 148, 201, 202

ALZHEIMER'S, 19, 47, 49, 82, 83, 84, 178, 179

AMERICAN DIET, SEE WESTERN DIET

AMINO ACIDS, 75, 87, 90, 98, 113, 123, 125

ANEMIA, 21, 23, 57, 79, 126

ANTIBIOTIC, 4, 25, 41, 60, 85, 86, 120, 121

ANTI-INFLAMMATORY, SEE INFLAM-MATION

ANTIOXIDANT, 23, 26, 49, 53, 55, 56, 76, 81, 82, 84, 87, 88, 89, 90, 93, 96, 97, 106, 110, 114, 124, 129, 140, 152, 153, 155, 156, 157

ANXIETY, 4, 41, 170

ARAME, 136, 139, 141, 145

ARTHRITIS, 44, 47, 52, 76, 77, 79, 114, 142, 170, 207

ASTAXANTHIN, 48, 152, 153, 154, 155, 156, 157, 158

ASTHMA, 44, 47, 65, 66, 67, 79, 142, 160

AUTISM, 96, 97

AUTOIMMUNE DISEASE, 44, 47, 142

AYURVEDA, 36, 46, 125

BARLEY/BARLEY GRASS, 12, 35, 64, 65, 66, 69, 73, 74, 78, 79, 81, 129, 130, 131, 160, 199

BEETS/BEET GREENS, 14, 60, 109, 124, 125, 126, 148

BETA-CAROTENE, SEE CAROTENE

BIOSPHERE II, 16

BIRD FLU, 60, 187, 193, 194

BLOCK, KEITH, 43, 92

BLOOD PRESSURE/HYPERTENSION, 12, 41, 44, 92, 124, 139, 189

BLOOD SUGAR, 63, 66, 76, 83, 93, 117, 129, SEE ALSO DIABETES

BLUE BERRIES, 48

BOK CHOY, 14, 105, 116

BRASSICA VEGETABLES, 104, 105, 109, 114

BROCCOLI/BROCCOLI SPROUTS, 13, 14, 30, 56, 103, 104, 105, 106, 109, 110, 111, 113, 114, 119, 128, 148, 197, 200

BRUSSELS SPROUTS, 30, 104, 105, 113

CABBAGE, 30, 60, 72, 104, 105, 106, 107, 108, 109, 110, 111, 112, 113, 119, 128, 147, 148, 200

CALCIUM, 52, 56, 57, 106, 117, 119, 120, 122, 124, 128, 135, 143, 144, 151, 161, 162, 163

CANCER, 4, 8, 13, 19, 20, 21, 22, 26, 28, 29, 31, 32, 43, 44, 49, 53, 54, 55, 58, 59, 61, 63, 67, 76, 77, 78, 82, 83, 91, 92, 101, 102, 105, 109, 110, 111, 112, 114, 115, 117, 118, 120, 121, 122, 124, 127, 129, 138, 139, 140, 141, 142, 169, 170, 179, 207

CANDIDA ALBICANS, 150

CANNABIS, SEE ALSO HEMP, SEE ALSO MARIJUANA, 169, 170, 171, 172, 173, 174, 175, 176, 177, 178, 179, 180, 191

CARDIOVASCULAR/HEART HEALTH, 82, 84, 88, 91, 92, 115, 124, 129

CAROTENE, 72, 87, 99, 106, 110, 114, 115, 116, 120, 124, 127, 128, 143, 153, 155, SEE ALSO VITAMIN A

CAROTENOIDS, 87, 117, 143, 156

CAULIFLOWER, 30, 104, 105, 106, 109, 111, 112, 113

CELIAC DISEASE, 64, 65, 73

CEREAL GRASSES, 12, 61, 63, 65, 66, 68, 70, 73, 76, 78, 80, 130

CHERRIES, 48, 199

CHICKEN POX, 149

CHLORELLA, 61, 79, 85, 86, 87, 88, 89, 90, 91, 92, 93, 94, 95, 96, 97, 98, 100, 136, 143, 148, 151, 160

CHLOROPHYLL, 10, 11, 15, 16, 17, 18, 19, 20, 23, 24, 25, 26, 27, 28, 29, 30, 31, 32, 38, 52, 64, 80, 87, 89, 98, 100, 122, 123, 128, 134, 143, 147, 148, 160

CHOLESTEROL, 7, 12, 17, 41, 43, 44, 48, 49, 83, 84, 89, 92, 117, 129, 152

COLDS/FLU, 70, 85, 86, 92, 95, 101, 138, 151, 187, 198, 193, 194, 195

COLITIS, 20, 21, 66, 170
    ULCERATIVE, 66, 76, 93, 94, SEE ALSO GASTROINTESTI-NAL HEALTH

COLLARD GREENS, 116, 119

COLONY COLLAPSE DISORDER (CCD), 185, 186

CRUCIFERS, 116

CURCUMIN, 83, 111, 112

DEPRESSION, 44, 177

DETOXIFICATION, 19, 26, 31, 55, 56, 76, 80, 84, 88, 89, 90, 91, 94, 96, 97, 110, 120, 128, 204, 208, SEE ALSO TOXINS

DIABETES, 7, 13, 21, 41, 44, 54, 63, 93, 116, 129, 170, 207, SEE ALSO BLOOD SUGAR

DNA, 14, 31, 48, 49, 62, 77, 78, 80, 90, 111, 114, 129, 150, 152, 155, 158

DULSE, 131, 134, 135, 136, 139, 141, 142, 145, 201

EBOLA, 187, 188, 189, 190, 191

ECZEMA, 21, 44, 108, SEE ALSO SKIN HEALTH

ENERGY FIELDS, 161, 164, 167

ENZYMES, 14, 23, 27, 31, 45, 53, 54, 55, 56, 59, 60, 62, 64, 68, 75, 80, 85, 89, 100, 106, 109, 110, 111, 122, 127, 128, 129, 130, 152, 160

ESTROGEN, 55, 110, 128, 141
        PHYTOESTROGENS, 128, 141
        XENOESTROGENS, 141

EXTINCTION, 2, 3

EYE HEALTH, 115, 117, 152

FATIGUE, 4, 5, 22, 51, 61, 79, 81, 95, 126, 189

FATTY ACIDS, 13, 123, 156, 158

FERMENTATION, 59, 60, 132

FERTILITY/INFERTILITY, 3, 25, 70, SEE ALSO REPRODUCTIVE HEALTH

FIBER, 4, 27, 59, 87, 88, 94, 104, 107, 110, 115, 117, 127, 134, 138, 139, 140, 142, 151, 152, 155, 160, 172, 201, 203

FIBROMYALGIA, 22, 95, 170

FOLIC ACID, 14, 110, 114, 115

GASTROINTESTINAL (GI) HEALTH, 13, 19, 29, 64, 65, 107, 137, 140, 142, SEE ALSO COLITIS; IRRITABLE BOWEL SYNDROME

GENETICALLY MODIFIED ORGAN-ISMS (GMOS), 3, 4, 147, 161, 181, 182, 183, 184, 187

GREEN TEA, 82, 83, 84, 121, 202

GREEN TEA SEED OIL, 48, 82, 83, 202, 203

GUM HEALTH, 23

HEADACHES, 20, 61, 66, 108

HEART HEALTH, SEE CARDIOVASCU-LAR HEALTH

HEAVY METALS, 80, 83, 88, 91, 142, 151

HEMP, 169, 172, 173, 175, SEE ALSO CANNABIS; MARIJUANA

HERPES (HSV), 41, 85, 101, 138, 144, 149, 150, 151

HIJIKI, 134, 135, 136, 139, 141, 145, 201

HIV, 101, 138, 177, 190, 191, 192, SEE ALSO AIDS

HIPPOCRATES INSTITUTE, 21, 23, 160

HYDRILLA, 135, 143, 144

HYPERTENSION, SEE BLOOD PRES-SURE

IMMUNE HEALTH, 4, 30, 43, 47, 48, 76, 90, 91, 92, 93, 95, 100, 101, 102, 110, 114, 121, 124, 125, 126, 129, 138, 149, 150, 151, 156, 179, 186, 187, 189, 190, 191, 201

INFLAMMATION/ANTI-INFLAMMA-TORY, 45, 47, 62, 63, 82, 83, 94, 100, 142, 149, 156, 158, 170, 171

IRON, 23, 24, 57, 100, 112, 122, 124

IRRITABLE BOWEL SYNDROME, 32, 65, 118, SEE ALSO GASTRO-INTESTI-NAL HEALTH

KALE, 11, 14, 27, 104, 105, 109, 116, 117, 118, 119, 125, 128, 200

KAMUT, 1, 2, 29, 65, 66, 73, 74, 79, 81

KELP, 135, 136, 137, 138, 139, 140, 141, 142, 145

KIDNEY HEALTH, 14, 50, 198

KOMBU, 145

LEGUMES, 35, 39, 59, 127, 129, 130, 183, 197, 203

LIFE-FIELDS (L-FIELDS), 166, 167, SEE ALSO ENERGY FIELDS

LIVER HEALTH, 21, 23, 26, 31, 55, 56, 75, 80, 84, 89, 90, 93, 111, 116, 125, 126, 128, 170

MAGNESIUM, 19, 20, 57, 87, 100, 122, 135, 138, 143, 161, 163

MARIJUANA, 168, 169, 170, 171, 172, 173, 174, 175, 176, 177, 178, 179, 180, SEE ALSO CANNABIS; HEMP

MUSTARD GREENS, 14

NIES, ERIC, 6

NORI, 131, 134, 135, 136, 139, 145

OBESITY, 5, 12, 21, 27, 63, 83, 93, 123, 134, 138, 156, 195

OXIDATION, 45, 48, 49, 56, 57, 83, 93, 106, 158

PERTUSSIS/WHOOPING COUGH, 86

PH, 29, 49, 50, 51, 52, 53

PHYCOCYANINS, 99, 100

PLANT BASED NUTRITION PRO-GRAM/PLAN, 57, 42, 79, 96

POMEGRANATE, 201

POTASSIUM, 52, 106, 119, 121, 122, 124, 144, 163

PREGNANCY, 57, 115, 191

PROBIOTICS, 27, 60, 94, 97

RAW FOODS, 20, 21, 49, 56, 66, 67, 81

REJUVELAC, 130, 131, 132

REPRODUCTIVE HEALTH, 61, SEE ALSO FERTILITY/INFERTILITY

RESPIRATORY HEALTH, 47, 50, 51, 92, 108

RESVERATROL, 83

SCHNABEL, CHARLES, 70, 72, 80

SEAWEED, 17, 120, 131, 134, 135, 136, 137, 138, 139, 140, 141, 142, 144, 145, 149

SEEDS, 13, 20, 34, 39, 59, 64, 67, 73, 82, 83, 105, 109, 112, 116, 118, 125, 127, 130, 131, 132, 145, 163, 169, 203

SINUS HEALTH, 17, 22, 26, 44, 63

SKIN HEALTH, 99, 153, SEE ALSO ACNE; ECZEMA

SPINACH, 14, 32, 72, 81, 115, 122, 123, 124, 125, 126, 128

SPIRULINA, 37, 79, 81, 85, 87, 98, 99, 100, 101, 102, 136, 148, 198

SPROUTS, 14, 20, 30, 64, 103, 104, 105, 109, 110, 113, 126, 127, 128, 129, 130, 131, 132, 163

SUBTLE ORGANIZING ENERGY FIELDS (SOFES), SEE ENERGY FIELDS

SUPEROXIDE DISMUTASE (SOD), 54, 56, 76, 77, 155

SWISS CHARD, 124, 126

TOXINS, 4, 31, 46, 55, 58, 60, 62, 77, 78, 80, 88, 89, 94, 105, 126, 137, 138, 140, 142, 198, SEE ALSO DETOXIFICATION

TRACE MINERALS, 9, 45, 52, 56, 57, 100, 104, 184, 204

TRADITIONAL CHINESE MEDICINE (TCM), 46

TRIGLYCERIDES, 43, 129

TURMERIC, 83, 111, 112

TURNIP/TURNIP GREENS, 60, 104, 105, 125

VITAMIN A, 23, 37, 72, 87, 110, 114, 115, 116, SEE ALSO CAROTENE

VITAMIN B1, 106

VITAMIN B12, 139, 144

VITAMIN B2/RIBOFLAVIN, 106, 122, 140

VITAMIN C, 60, 72, 87, 106, 110, 114, 117, 120, 122, 126, 128, 143, 153

VITAMIN D, 37, 57

VITAMIN D3, 57

VITAMIN E, 23, 106, 153

VITAMIN K, 23, 107, 117

VITAMIN U, 107

WAKAME, 135, 136, 139, 145, 201

WATERCRESS, 163

WESTERN DIET/AMERICAN DIET, 23, 35, 94, 125, 133, 134, 140

WHEATGRASS, 2, 20, 21, 31, 64, 65, 66, 67, 68, 73, 74, 75, 76, 78, 79, 160

WIGMORE, ANN, 14, 20, 21, 23, 31, 75, 76, 79, 130, 131, 132, 160, 206

YARBROUGH, MANNY (TINY), 5, 6, 7, 207

ZINC, 56, 57, 119

# SPECIAL DEDICATION

The final thoughts go to the person that I owe the greatest thanks for my success in pursuing my dreams, the person who somehow came along with my vision, despite hardships and stresses that few are willing to endure in pursuit of making the world a better place. And although the journey was much more difficult than we ever imagined and it seemed that at times the stress had all but destroyed us, the purpose and philosophy we are guided by was bigger than either of us and ultimately carried us through. So to Amy, for the hours and the years, the blood, sweat, and tears, I will care for you... always and forever.

# ABOUT THE AUTHOR

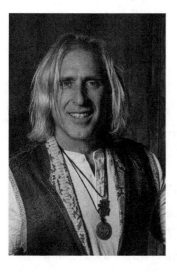

Dave Sandoval literally wrote the book on green foods nutrition. His book "The Green Foods Bible" has been translated into 4 languages and is the definitive guide to all the best green superfoods from the land and the sea. Despite Sandoval's many successes and high profile within and outside of the industry, his beginnings were altruistic and humble in nature. After watching loved ones suffer from (and sometimes succumb to) the ravages of preventable diseases, Sandoval decided to devote his life to making a difference in the health of others. He has spent many years combining scientific research and traditional holistic teachings from around the world to compose dozens of phytonutrient-rich formulas with the painstaking selection of only the most pure and premium ingredients. As owner of Purium Health Products, he feels blessed to bring the gift of health to millions of people around the globe.

"Our mission at Purium is simple – we want to help you eat better, age more gracefully and live longer." – David Sandoval

David Sandoval was born in Southern California and lived a meager existence for most of his young life. At the age of 17 he was forever changed by the tragic, untimely death of his favorite aunt who had taken him in off the streets and given him a home. Knowing that the cause of her illness was a poor diet and chemically-treated processed food, he eagerly studied all means of natural healing and chose to apply what he had learned from Ann Wigmore, the mother of the "Living Foods Lifestyle," into his own life.

What began as a quest to save the health of his family members became a passion to help families throughout the world.

David has dedicated his life to providing whole food, raw food, green food products with absolutely no artificial colors, artificial flavors, binders, fillers or genetically-modified ingredients. He quickly became recognized for setting a new standard for purity, potency, and cutting edge Plant- Based Nutritional Products that retain the vital essence (AKA life force, chi, or prana) that he believes is the key to fueling our cells.

For more than 20 years, David has researched and studied alongside the most recognized industry leaders from around the world … advancing his knowledge, creating new formulations and NEVER compromising on the ingredients and products that come from his facility.

His audio lecture CD, *The Healing Miracle of Green Foods* has now been translated into many languages and hundreds of thousands of copies have been distributed worldwide. His best-selling book *The Green Foods Bible* has also been translated into several languages and is a green super food resource that no home should be without.